HEARING AND THE HOSPITAL

First published in 2013 by
Sean Kingston Publishing
www.seankingston.co.uk
Canon Pyon

British Library Cataloguing in Publication Data
A catalogue record for this book is available from the British Library.

Printed by Lightning Source

ISBN 978-1-907774-24-9

Hearing and the Hospital

Sound, listening, knowledge and experience

Tom Rice

Sean Kingston Publishing
www.seankingston.co.uk
Canon Pyon

For Paul

CONTENTS

Introduction		1
Chapter 1	**Soundselves** *Sound, Surveillance and Selfhood on Hospital Wards*	21
Chapter 2	**Broadcasting the Body** *The Private Made Public in Hospital Soundscapes*	38
Chapter 3	**Acoustemology of the Body** *A Brief History of Diagnostic Listening*	55
Chapter 4	**'The Hallmark of a doctor'** *The Stethoscope and the Making of Medical Identity*	72
Chapter 5	**Learning to Listen** *Auscultation and the Transmission of Auditory Knowledge*	92
Chapter 6	**'Beautiful Murmurs'** *Stethoscopic Listening and Acoustic Objectification*	116
Chapter 7	**Auto-auscultation** *Listening to the Self*	137
Chapter 8	**Deathoscope** *Auscultation, Echocardiography and the 'Death of the Stethoscope'*	153
Conclusion		171
Appendix	**The Doctor**	184
References		189
Index		200

LIST OF FIGURES

Figure 1	Blind doctor Albert-Andre Nast using his ear instead of a stethoscope.	59
Figure 2	The Traditional Sprague.	84
Figure 3	The Harvey Triple Head.	85
Figure 4	A simple diagram of the heart.	97
Figure 5	Key listening points for cardiac auscultation.	101
Figure 6	Heart murmur sketches.	104
Figure 7	A teaching stethoscope.	106
Figure 8	A phonocardiogram of the murmur of mitral regurgitation.	108
Figure 9	An amplified stethoscope.	112

ACKNOWLEDGEMENTS

This book is based on three years of doctoral research made possible by an Economic and Social Research Council Ph.D. Studentship. I was also fortunate to receive an Economic and Social Research Council Postdoctoral Research Fellowship which gave me the opportunity to develop and consolidate the text. I am hugely grateful to my Postdoctoral Supervisor, Georgina Born, who has always been encouraging and generous with her time, giving careful readings and providing helpful and insightful comments on numerous drafts. I would also like to thank my Ph.D. supervisors, Sophie Day and Simon Cohn, who shaped and gave direction to the research in its early stages.

It has been inspiring to be able to have conversations during the project with some of those whose work has defined the recent academic enthusiasm for 'sound studies'. I am grateful to Tia DeNora, John Drever, John Wynne, Steven Feld, Don Brenneis, Karin Bijsterveld, Peter Cusack, Angus Carlyle, Cathy Lane, Stephanie Bunn, David Toop, Marina Roseman, Les Back and Tim Ingold, who all showed interest in the research.

I would like to thank the members of the Edinburgh Hospital Broadcasting Service for giving me the initial opportunity to study the sounds of a hospital, and Dr John Coltart for making it possible for me to conduct fieldwork at the Cardiothoracic Unit at St Thomas'. His open-mindedness and sustained enthusiasm for the project has been invaluable. I am also particularly grateful to the first group of medical students I encountered during fieldwork: Rishi Caleyachetty, Tom Simpson, Sue Ann Knight, Dave Tang, Harjit Bhogal, Mary Anandarajah, Diane Sivnort and Alistair Matthews. They made me feel welcome from the first day and made the entire year fun. The stethoscope, which has linked together so many doctors and patients, has also connected many friends. I owe special thanks to Douglas Rice for proof reading the text and to Alison Rice, Paul Strauss and Anna Glayzer, all of whom have been hugely supportive. Finally, thanks to Kate Taunton, for sharing the process and shining her positivity on it all.

'Listening must be examined – itself auscultated' (Jean-Luc Nancy)

INTRODUCTION

This book is an ethnographic study of some of the different forms of listening practised in two hospitals at which I conducted research between 1999 and 2004. These were the Edinburgh Royal Infirmary in Edinburgh, Scotland, and St Thomas' Hospital in London, England. It focuses first on patients' experiences of the sonic environments that characterise hospital wards, and briefly considers the monitory listening practised by nurses as they manage patients on wards. The book goes on to examine ways in which sound and listening are also used in diagnostic work, exploring in particular the practice of stethoscopic listening or auscultation as learned and performed by medical students and doctors. The hospital is shown to be a space in which several modes of listening are simultaneously in play, and in which different layers of auditory knowledge and experience coexist. While for the purposes of clarity it is helpful to differentiate the types of listening practised by patients, nurses and doctors in order to make comparisons possible, the book also draws attention to certain contexts in which these modes of auditory attention and the perspectives they confer can merge, interact or inform one another.

As an anthropological study, the book attempts to show how sound and listening produce, articulate and mediate social relations inside the hospital. Differentiating between the listening practices of patients, nurses and doctors suggests that what a person listens to, and what he or she hears or is able to hear, is an expression of his or her social position in the hospital, a marker of his or her relative knowledge, skill and power. The book does indeed engage with listening practices as markers of social difference, and as channels through which the social hierarchy of the hospital is produced and reproduced. At the same time, however, it positions listening as a form of experience that is shaped and moulded by social context, paying close attention to the ways in which auditory capacities acquire direction and focus, and in which sounds become endowed with particular meanings and associations within the cultural environment that the hospital represents.

Ironically, I think it is partly because hospital listening practices are often so ubiquitous, and seem so trivial compared to the more dramatic activities and events that take place within hospitals, that they deserve and indeed necessitate study. They can easily be overlooked. A patient's reactions to noise on the ward, for instance, might seem to be of little consequence compared to, say, the success of his or her surgery. Yet patients can spend long periods of time, often confined to bed, exposed to the sounds of the people and practices around them. Some medical professionals have (rightly in my view) expressed concern that excessive and largely preventable noise on wards might negatively affect patient health and recovery times (e.g. Bharathan *et al.* 2007). The term 'noise', though, can lead us to think somewhat reductively, dwelling on notions of irritation and annoyance, overlooking the more complex meanings and associations that ward sounds can hold for those who are immersed in them. In part, this book attempts to tease out some of the detail of patient responses to the sounds to which they are obliged to listen on hospital wards. It also examines how particular acoustic phenomena can have a powerful bearing on patients' wider experiences of illness and of hospitalization.

In a similar way, professional listening practices are often routine and commonplace. They may lack the heroics of surgery or the technological cachet of, for instance, nuclear imaging. However, a consideration of the intricacies of how listening is used and applied within the hospital exposes some of the sensory minutiae that both underpin and undermine the production of medical knowledge and skill. Modes of auditory attention might be understood to have developed as responses to challenges in diagnosis or patient management, yet they are also expressions of ideologies and attitudes which, while possessing rich histories, continue to inform and structure contemporary clinical work. At the same time, some listening techniques are shown to have acquired significance that far exceeds their apparent practical value, being bound up in some cases with strongly emotive debates about how medicine should be practised. Importantly, reflecting on medical listening also invites a re-appraisal of ideas and assumptions about the nature of the sense of hearing, and how it may be used and applied. It creates scope for a re-evaluation of the perceptual possibilities of audition itself.

Research background

My interest in hospital listening began when, as an undergraduate in Social Anthropology at the University of Edinburgh, I was required to write a dissertation on a subject of my own choosing based on three months of ethnographic research. At this time I was working as a volunteer for *Red Dot Radio*, the Edinburgh Hospital Broadcasting Service. The service broadcast to patients inside the Infirmary, as it still does at the time of writing, between 7 and 10 p.m. each evening. Patients were able to listen to the output through headphones attached to a socket in the wall beside their beds.

My main job at the station was to visit the wards to talk to patients, gather feedback about previous shows and obtain music requests. The station seemed to have a large number of regular listeners amongst medium- and long-term patients in particular. As I went about my work it became apparent that one of the key reasons patients chose to listen to the station was that it gave them an opportunity to escape from the sounds of the ward. In fact, some would lie in bed with the headphones on even when there was no music playing in an attempt to block out the noise around them. For many patients, the sounds of the ward were a distinctive feature of life in hospital (Rice 2003, 2008a). Surprised by the intensity of patient feeling about the sonic environment, I chose to devote my fieldwork period and subsequent dissertation to exploring patients' acoustic experiences of hospital wards. Insights from this initial research period inform the first two chapters of this book in particular.

This early piece of ethnographic fieldwork involved my visiting patients on a wide range of wards. On the cardiology wards especially, however, I noticed doctors listening to patients' chests using stethoscopes. The stethoscope allowed them, it seemed, almost completely to exclude the noise of the ward and immerse themselves instead in sounds from patients' bodies. As I had become aware of patient understandings of ward sounds, watching this practice made me conscious that different modes of listening, types of acoustic knowledge and acoustic perspectives could be found on the wards. At the same time, observing auscultation brought about the realization that the body could be understood as an 'acoustic space' of which doctors had a specialized appreciation (Carpenter and McLuhan 1960:65). The tones of machines used to monitor the activity of the heart were also noticeable on these wards, and made events inside the body audibly intelligible to health professionals. Listening practices, it seemed, were varied and intense in cardiology.

I did not immediately seek to develop my initial study of hospital listening further. After finishing my undergraduate degree I went to the University of Manchester to pursue a postgraduate course in Visual Anthropology. During that year I developed a slight chest infection and went to see a local GP (General Practitioner). He listened to my chest with a stethoscope, and I remember feeling that he seemed to be taking a considerable amount of time over it. 'Ah yes,' he said presently, 'you most definitely have a heart murmur.' It turned out that the murmur was very slight, and did not pose a threat to my general health. However, I was horrified to learn of it, and at the same time intrigued by the way the sound inside my body had been detected and interpreted by the listening doctor. The interaction renewed my interest in the body as an acoustic space, in the auditory knowledge that doctors bring to the investigation of its sounds and in the experience of those who are recipients of or made subject to medical listening practices. Indeed, it could be argued that this book represents a gigantic hypochondriac indulgence.

I assembled a Ph.D. proposal and in due course enrolled at Goldsmiths College, University of London. Because of my awareness of the potential diagnostic significance of heart sounds, and having noted the intensive use of cardiac auscultation on the cardiology wards at the Edinburgh Royal Infirmary, I decided to focus on the medical practice of listening to the heart. Searching for a fieldwork site, I wrote to Dr John Coltart, Director of the specialist Cardiothoracic Unit at St Thomas' Hospital in Waterloo, London. The research proposal interested him because he had long been conscious of the importance of listening in his everyday practice. He said he considered his ears to be one of his most important clinical tools, and, as he had been teaching auscultation for a long time, was interested in the qualities that made students 'good listeners'. Dr Coltart agreed to support my application for Honorary Observer status within Guy's and St Thomas' hospital. This unpaid position would enable me to observe any clinical interactions that took place there. I would be authorized to sit in on consultations, ward rounds, and even operations provided I sought permission from patients and the staff in charge of their care. Dr Coltart also suggested I participate in classes for medical students, and it was this which ultimately formed the backbone of my research.

So in October 2003 I returned to St Thomas' for a year-long placement. The job title, it turned out, was not one many people at the hospital had come across. Though being an Honorary Observer gave me less authority even than the medical students with whom I began working, it sounded prestigious, and throughout my year of fieldwork if I asked permission to attend, for instance, a ward round, I was never refused. Dr Coltart allowed me to accompany him to his clinics and the classes he taught, and introduced me to the other doctors, the medical students and nurses whose voices are present within this book. My observations made through learning auscultation form the basis of Chapters 3–8. However, this second period of research also represented an opportunity to widen and deepen my understanding of patient perceptions of the sonic environments of hospital wards. It allowed me, too, to develop a sense of how medical modes of listening differed or were connected, and how they fitted into the wider sensory economy of the hospital. Dr Coltart was my first point of contact at St Thomas' and acted as my supervisor there.

He is frequently quoted in what follows. Like John Berger's (1967) account of the life of Dr John Sassall, and Robert Hahn's (1985) study of internist Dr Barry Seigler, my work is flavoured by respect for the work of the man who is arguably its key protagonist, by gratitude for his support and enthusiasm, and by a straightforward liking of the man himself.

The 'rotation' and the 'firm'

As Dr Coltart had suggested, it seemed that teaching sessions would be a promising juncture at which to access the particular kind of auditory knowledge which auscultation represents. Teaching would involve senior doctors explaining the skill to medical students. The technique would be in the process of transmission, its subtleties and secrets being made plain for the novice. I would be able to explore the pedagogical techniques used by teaching doctors to communicate aspects of auscultation, and examine the manner in which the students were influenced by the acquisition of new perceptual and diagnostic powers.

The time required to become a qualified doctor in the UK depends on the route a person takes through the education system and the structure of the particular course on which he or she is enrolled. At the time my research took place, however, medical training was generally expected to take five years. Teaching during the first two years (known as the 'pre-clinical' or sometimes the 'pre-cynical' years) mostly took place in the classroom and involved lectures and tutorials, with assessments in the form of written exercises and exams. The emphasis was on anatomy and on the necessary aspects of chemistry and biology for understanding the constitution, function, and treatment of the body within a Western medical framework. On completion of this pre-clinical training, students would undertake three 'clinical years', mainly focused on supervised contact with patients on hospital wards. It was in the first of these years that students were introduced to auscultation, and I therefore focused my fieldwork on groups of third year medical students who were learning to listen for the first time.

St Thomas' Hospital, and Guy's Hospital which is located nearby on the south side of the Thames at London Bridge, are run by a single managing trust, the Guy's and St Thomas' NHS (National Health Service) Foundation Trust. In 1998 these two hospitals became linked to a third hospital, King's Hospital in Denmark Hill, South London. They pooled their academic resources to form Guy's, King's and St Thomas' Medical School, also known as GKT. In late 2005 GKT was re-named the King's College London School of Medicine and Dentistry at Guy's, King's College and St Thomas' Hospitals, usually referred to as the King's College London School of Medicine.

The students with whom I began studying in 2003 were all GKT students who were just beginning their first year of clinics. The year's practical teaching was subdivided into three 'rotations', each of which focused on one particular area of the body: the abdomen, head or chest. Each rotation lasted for three months, with several tuition sessions each week. The group of between five and ten students assigned to each rotation was called a 'firm'; they were together for the twelve weeks of a rotation. At the beginning of my fieldwork I joined a firm of students just starting their first rotation, which for them was the 'chest rotation'. In the course of my research I became close to this group. Its members are often quoted in the book and so I introduce them by name here: Tom, Sue Ann, Dave, Diane, Harjit, Alistair, Rishi and Mary. All were between the ages of twenty and twenty-three during the research period, and are now qualified doctors.

The anthropology of the senses

The development of this book has been strongly influenced by the 'anthropology of the senses', a sub-discipline that began to emerge formally in the 1980s and 90s out of an earlier wave of anthropological interest in embodiment (Howes 1991a:3–4, Pink 2009:11). The fundamental premise of the anthropology of the senses or 'sensorial anthropology' is that sensory perception is a cultural as well as a physical act (Howes 1991b:167). That is, the senses are not only mechanistic receptors of information but are also mediators of social value. The value accorded to types of sensory experience varies historically and cross-culturally. Howes, perhaps the scholar most active in outlining a remit for the anthropology of the senses, suggests that the task of the sensory anthropologist is to examine the particular way in which a given society configures the senses and invests different sensory domains with social value. Thus, the anthropology of the senses is 'primarily concerned with how the patterning of sense experience varies from one culture to the next in accordance with the meaning and emphasis attached to each of the modalities of perception' (1991a:3).

The patterning of the senses evident in a culture produces a distinctive 'sensory profile' belonging to that culture (Carpenter 1976:28, Howes and Classen 1991:257). Picking up the concept of a 'ratio among the senses' (see McLuhan [1962] 2008:88, Ong 1991), Howes ventures that societies tend to order the senses hierarchically, with one sense often accorded priority over the others. Howes' (1988) work on olfactory classification in Eastern Indonesia and Western Melanesia, for instance, leads him to distinguish between odour-accepting and odour-denying societies. He identifies a complex vocabulary of olfactory terms for the description of people and behaviours, and points to ways in which, particularly among the societies of the Tanimbar Islands and

New Caledonia, smells are integral to local cosmology, to perceptions of the living and the dead, and to notions of transition between life and death. Here the sense of smell is privileged in the sensory order in ways in which it is not elsewhere.

Like others, Howes characterizes Western society as a visual society (e.g. Classen 1998, Stoller 1989, 1997, Tyler 1984). He makes reference to the visual foundations of Western knowledge and aesthetics, noting a 'long-established Western bias in favour of sight' (1991a:10). This bias is considered to have pervaded Western scholarship, including anthropology, which in his view lacks a truly multisensory orientation, as a consequence of which it is not only impoverished but is also frequently inaccurate in its engagement with and representation of other cultures. Howes argues that anthropologists must develop 'a rigorous awareness of the visual and textual biases of the Western episteme' (ibid.:3). Only then can we 'hope to make sense of how life is lived in other cultural settings' (ibid.). His advocating the anthropology of the senses reflects a desire to celebrate the non-visual senses in particular, reawakening academics to the multiplicity of sensory possibilities and drawing attention to the manner in which alternative sensory realities are lived by others. This call is echoed in the work of Stoller (1997), who urges a sensory reinvigoration of ethnographic research and writing, advocating what he calls a 'sensuous scholarship'.

Following my initial period of ethnography in particular, I found this formative outlining of the anthropology of the senses helpful. At a time when few people (and certainly none of my supervisors) were working on sound within anthropology, it legitimized my focus on sensory experience and provided a (sub)-disciplinary home for my research. Indeed, this book as a whole continues to speak to core concerns within the anthropology of the senses. Most fundamentally, it asserts the relevance of sensory and specifically sonic meaning to ethnographic enquiry. It also represents an ethnographic attempt to explore the lived sensory worlds of (albeit Western) others.

The anthropology of the senses is, at the time of writing, an active and productive sub-discipline (Bull and Back 2003a, Classen 2005, Korsmeyer 2005, Drobnik 2006, Edwards and Bhaumik 2008, Howes 2009). The underpinnings of the anthropology of the senses have received criticism, however, and these criticisms have in turn had a formative influence on this book. Ingold (2000), for instance, makes the point that Howes' emphasis on a society's conceptualization and hierarchical valuation of the senses leads to a tendency to overlook the importance of lived sensory experience and the manner in which meaning is generated by individuals through actual acts and practices of looking, listening and so on. Thus, rather than positioning the senses as abstract categories, or socially imposed perceptual schemes, Ingold advocates closer attention to the manner in which the individual's 'sensory capacities are practically deployed in activities of perception' (ibid.:285). This book responds to Ingold's appeal for close attention to the specificities of sensory practice. The auditory skills and acuities of medical students and doctors, it suggests, are formed not by virtue of a kind of conformism to a particular sensory model, but through practical apprenticeship within a professional community. At the same time, patients' engagements with ward sounds are not rigidly culturally predetermined, but constitute an ongoing set of responses to the clinical environment in which they find themselves. However, I have found it important not to lose sight of the outline of the anthropology of the senses provided by Howes. The material that follows illustrates, for instance, that different values may be placed on auditory and visual evidence in Western medicine, and that these different valuations have important implications in relation to how both resources and faith are invested in diagnostic technology. The book therefore attempts to maintain sensitivity to the manner in which different sensory domains and practices may be invested with social value.

Serematakis describes the notion of sensory ratios or balances that appears fundamental to Howes' programme for the anthropology of the senses as a 'vital analytic lens of the comparative approach' (1994b:126). However, she is wary of efforts to enumerate sensory capacities and delimit zones of experience, which, she suggests, although potentially allowing additional or alternative categories, are nonetheless liable to constitute 'an objectifying grid that distorts or effaces the manner in which a culture senses the senses' (ibid.). Serematakis prefers to regard the senses as fluid 'semantic currents' (1994a:5). Her work focuses on the manner in which sensory experiences transform and are transformed through processes of memory and imagination. As both Serematakis and Stoller point out, it does indeed seem nonsensical to adopt an approach that overlooks the fact that the members of any society use all of their senses in overlapping and integrated ways. Indeed, hearing in the medical setting is often used and applied in close interplay with the other senses (Rice 2007) and a recurring theme throughout this book is the manner in which the senses of hearing and sight, while at times polarized and placed in opposition to one another, are often tightly linked through both metaphor and practice in medical work. At the same time, though, while responsive to Serematakis's assertion of the need for sensitivity to fluidity and interplay between the senses, I am conscious of the need at times to redraw boundaries between sensory categories in order to keep sound and listening at the centre of the analysis, and in order to be able to keep relationships between modes of perception clear.

While attacking the conceptual framework of the anthropology of the senses proposed by Howes, criticisms such as these from Ingold and Serematakis have ultimately, I would argue, enriched and expanded the scope of an 'anthropology of the senses' rather than invalidating it as an approach or an area of study. They have demonstrated the potential for a range of critical and theoretical positions to both co-exist within and contribute to a sensorial anthropology. The critiques all fundamentally restate the importance for anthropologists of reflection on the nature of the senses and on their involvement in social life.

Chuengsatiansup writes that '[i]n the anthropology of medicine, a new wave of ethnographic study has taken sensory experience to be a crucial aspect of medical phenomena' (1999:277). He points to the work of Daniel (1991), who examines the tactile examination of the pulse in diagnostic practice in Indian Siddha medicine (Hsu's 1999, 2010 work on pulse diagnostics in Chinese medicine is also relevant here). He also refers to descriptions by Classen *et al.* (1994) of the importance of the olfactory sense in a variety of healing rituals, and Desjarlais' (1992) work on the importance of the proprioceptive sense in activity surrounding the healing of 'soul loss' in the Nepalese Himalayas. Chuengsatiansup considers his own research to add to this growing body of work on the involvement of the senses in illness and suffering. He focuses on the close association between sound and a form of illness that affects a significant number of women in Kui communities in Northeastern Thailand. The illness is characterized by symptoms including sleeplessness, shortness of breath, feeling frightened, loss of appetite and chronic fatigue. While Chuengsatiansup acknowledges that several anthropological works focus on sonic experience and on the use of musical performances in healing rituals (e.g. Roseman 1991, Kleinman 1995, Friedson 1996, Laderman and Roseman 1996), his own work examines how the 'felt immediacies' of certain non-musical sounds occurring within everyday village life are 'reconceptualised within the indigenous somato-psychic framework as a form of illness' (1999:274).

Like Chuengsatiansup's work, this book seeks to contribute to a cross-fertilization of the anthropology of the senses and medical anthropology by providing a further ethnographic context in which non-musical, often banal sound forms become involved in illness experience. It not only considers patient responses to ward sounds, but also examines how patients' subjection to techniques of medical listening can lead them to report pronounced feelings of alienation and objectification. At the same time, patients' exposure to and interpretation of sounds produced by medical technologies can at times provoke disturbing kinds of introspection, initiating troubling speculation as to the origin and diagnostic significance of heard sounds. Admittedly, patients are in hospital because of existing health problems, so that their auditory experiences inside the institution cannot be linked, as they are in the Kui example, to initial symptoms or be regarded as the source of illness. Nonetheless, the book shows that sounds can become integral to patients' experiences of feeling and being ill.

In its discussion of cardiac auscultation, this book draws on a number of historical pieces (Reiser 1978, 1997, Porter 1997, Lachmund 1999, Sterne 2003a, 2003b, Nicolson 2004). These sources have been immensely valuable in helping me to understand how auscultation emerged and why it became integrated into routine medical practice in the West. This book attempts to complement these historical sources by providing an account of the practice in a contemporary medical setting, and by giving phenomenological detail of the experience of learning and using stethoscopic listening. In doing so, it aims to make an additional contribution to the overlapping spheres of medical anthropology and the anthropology of the senses by detailing the involvement of auditory knowledge and skill in the production and reproduction of medical knowledge.

As indicated above, Howes suggests that the senses are valued differently in different cultures, and that in any one culture a particular sense may come to be privileged as a sensory mode. Illustrating this concept he makes an extended reference to Stoller's (1989) work among the Songhay, one element of which concerns Stoller's apprenticeship to a sorcerer. Stoller is upbraided by his teacher, who reminds him of the importance of 'learning how to *hear*' if he is to gain real insight into Songhay ways (ibid.:115, original italics). Stoller details his gradual realization that comprehending the Songhay world would involve a number of sensory re-adjustments. For example, he came to recognize that the magical power of certain Songhay words lay not in their function as signifiers, but rather in their character as acoustic events and in the particular sonic energy they embodied and imparted (ibid.:115–22). Stoller was required to overcome his cultural verbocentrism and preoccupation with linguistic meaning and attune himself instead to the acoustic qualities and dynamics of vocalizations in Songhay sorcery. Howes considers Stoller's research to illustrate that for Songhay the world is 'constructed on an acoustic scaffolding…rather than a visual-spatial one, as in the West' (1991:10).

Further accounts of societies in which hearing is privileged as a sensory mode, and in which reality might be said to be constructed on 'an acoustic scaffolding', are provided by Feld in his ethnography on the Kaluli (1990, 1991, 1996, 2003), by Gell (1995) in his study of the Umeda, and by Weiner (1991) in his work on the Foi. These ethnographies, however, were carried out in the heartland of traditional anthropology, namely in rural, non-Western (and specifically, Papuan) contexts. This book, however, aims to provide a detailed consideration of practices of sonic knowing in an urban, Western, institutional setting. The hospital does not provide the sonic richness of the forest environments described by Feld, Gell and Weiner, nor do people living and working within the hospitals in which I conducted fieldwork practise and preserve such a complex set of cultural traditions relating to acoustic perception and interpretation. At the same time, aware of the constant assertion and reassertion of Western society as a visual culture, this study points to the hospital as an institution in which, while not necessarily dominant as a sensory mode, listening and auditory knowledge are of great importance. Also, while institutions have been the focus of much anthropological and sociological research, there has not yet, to my knowledge at least, been a detailed ethnography of sound based in an institution, let alone a hospital. This book therefore attempts to break new ethnographic ground.

Sound studies

Above, I identified important contributions to the anthropological study of sound, and indicated that these were a formative influence on the design of my own research (Stoller 1989, Feld 1990, 1991, 1996, 2003, Weiner 1991, Gell 1995). However, these texts (to which I return later) also represent the foundation of a burgeoning of interest in sound and listening within anthropology (e.g. Peek 1994, Ingold 2000, Feld and Brenneis 2004, Whitehouse 2006, Cox 2006, Hirschkind 2006, Helmreich 2007, Samuels *et al.* 2010). Erlmann makes reference to a 'resurgence of the ear', and I have argued elsewhere that there is a sufficient intellectual interest among anthropologists and ethnomusicologists, and a sufficiently substantial body of relevant work, to justify the recognition of 'auditory anthropology' as a legitimate sub-discipline (Erlmann 2004:2, Rice 2005).

The growth of interest in audition within anthropology has been matched by a corresponding profusion of work on sound and listening across other disciplines which, broadly speaking, 'share a recognition of the need for the cultural and historical contextualization of auditory perception' (Erlmann 2004:3). Among these often overlapping disciplines or areas of study are acoustic ecology and soundscape studies (e.g. Schafer 1977, Truax 1978), sociology (DeNora 2000, Back 2003, Beer 2010), history (B.R. Smith 1999, 2003, 2004, M.M. Smith 2001, 2004, Corbin 1998, Bailey 1996), archaeology (Watson and Keating 1999, Moore 2005), cultural geography (Rodaway 1994, Revill 2000, Matless 2005), science and technology studies (Pinch and Trocco 2002, Bijsterveld 2008, Pinch and Bijsterveld 2012a), communication studies (Truax 2001, Sterne 2003a, 2003b), media studies (Bull 2000), deaf studies (Bauman 2004, 2008), urban studies (Atkinson 2006, 2007), literature studies (Picker 2003, Connor 1997, 2000), sound art (Labelle 2010, Kahn 2001, Wynne 2007), film sound studies (Chion 1994, Lastra 2000) and theatre studies (Brown

2010). A strongly interdisciplinary academic field has therefore been created and has come to be known as 'sound studies' (Pinch and Bijsterveld 2004:636, 2012b:6–7). While this book is firmly embedded within anthropology, then, it both draws upon insights from, and develops discussions which it is hoped will be of interest to, academics and students working within sound studies more generally. Below I identify some major themes or areas of sound studies to which the book contributes.

Detailing the involvement of sound in establishing and articulating the distinctive character of the ward as an institutional medical space, the book connects with a large body of research that explores the relationship between sound and notions of space and place. It forges links, for instance, with Schafer's 'exemplary work on sound studies' in which, setting out the project of acoustic ecology, he introduces the term 'soundscape' and provides other key concepts and vocabulary for the description, mapping and analysis of sound environments (Pinch and Bijsterveld 2004:636, Schafer 1977). The book also responds to a loud call for careful consideration of the importance of sound in culturally particular experiences of place and emplacement (e.g. Feld 1996, Ingold 2000, Revill 2000, Matless 2005, Atkinson 2006, 2007). By examining the attempts made by patients to construct zones of privatized auditory space in a public environment, and exploring the constant reconfiguration of boundaries between professionalized and non-professionalized auditory spaces on the ward, the book also connects to core concerns in Bull's (2000) key sound studies work on personal stereo use and to themes in Corbin's (1998) important historical research on the use of bells in the marking and preservation of territory in nineteenth century France.

A feature of the 'aural architecture' of the hospital as experienced by many patients is the presence of unpleasant, unwanted and intrusive sounds (Blesser and Salter 2007). This book therefore works in parallel with a range of sources that explore noise as a cultural phenomenon and which examine the social and historical conditions within which certain sounds come to be identified as irritating, disturbing and unhealthy (e.g. Picker 2003, Thompson 2004, Bijsterveld 2003, 2008, Braun 2012). It also emphasizes that sound environments may have a powerful effect on human wellbeing, highlighting the importance of designing (in this case institutional) soundscapes so as improve them or preserve any positively experienced sonic qualities (e.g. Schafer 1977, Truax 1978).

In his major volume *The Audible Past*, Sterne (2003a) constructs a genealogy of sound reproduction technologies. He suggests that technologies only emerge within a wider cultural milieu that makes their production not only possible but also desirable. Considering auscultation, he suggests that the practice emerged as part of an 'Ensoniment' (which he argues took place contemporaneously and in conjunction with a wider Enlightenment) in which '[t]hrough techniques of listening, people harnessed, modified, and shaped their powers of auditory perception in the service of rationality' (ibid.:2). By discussing, like Sterne, the development of medical techniques of listening to the body and in particular the emergence of stethoscopic listening, this book reflects a concern in sound studies literature not only with exploring the ways in which people listened in the past (e.g. B.R. Smith 1999, 2003, 2004, M.M. Smith 2001, 2004, Corbin 1998, Bailey 1996), but also with tracing the origin and development of modern audio technologies and contemporary ways of listening (e.g. Pinch and Trocco 2002, Bijsterveld 2010, Fickers 2012). The book also contributes to the effort made by researchers within sound studies to show that listening is not a homogenous practice but takes a wide range of forms and involves a variety of modes of attention (e.g. Pinch and Bijsterveld 2012b:14, Truax 2001:21–31). Chapters outline several different types of listening that become evident on the hospital wards, specifying particular purposes and goals to which the sense of hearing has been applied. Like other sound studies work the book also explains how certain auditory aptitudes or sensitivities may be developed through training, becoming key and even definitive features of a professional skill set (Horning 2004, Porcello 2004, Krebs 2012).

Scholars working in the area of Science and Technology Studies (STS) have made a particularly strong contribution to sound studies, bringing to the fore the embeddedness of sound 'not only in history, society and culture, but also in science and technology and its machines and ways of knowing and interacting' (Pinch and Bijsterveld 2004:636). Researchers in STS have explored a wide variety of contexts in which sound and listening practices have been and continue to be involved in the generation of scientific knowledge, while attention has also been directed towards the interplay between sound, listening and technology in scientific work. This book speaks directly to STS work on sound, tracing the origins and development of auscultation as a mode of listening in the service of medical science and outlining the role that the technique continues to play in contemporary diagnostic practice. STS has also made the embodied connections between scientific practitioners and the tools they employ a focus of research, giving insight into 'the subtle interconnections between the experimenter's body, the use of scientific instruments, and the outcomes of laboratory work' (Pinch and Bijsterveld 2012b:13). This book pays careful attention to the detail of how auditory skills are formed and refined through a doctor's training and examines the close embodied familiarity with their stethoscopes that some doctors develop. Discussing the potential obsolescence of auscultation and its replacement by ultrasound imaging technology, the book also engages with another key theme of STS work on sound, namely attitudes towards listening techniques and questions over the epistemological status and legitimacy of sound in scientific practice (e.g. Supper 2012, Mody 2012).

Contributions to sound studies have both emphasized and demonstrated the value of sound and listening as rich sources of critical perspectives. An important aim of this book is to provide an acoustic interrogation of certain key concepts within anthropology and also social theory more widely, not seeking to discredit them but rather to augment their possibilities and potentials by considering them in what one might call an acoustic light. Thus, the book engages, for instance, with Foucault's (1973, 1977) discussions of disciplinary gazing and panopticism and with his work on the clinical gaze, exploring how reflections on sound and listening bring new dimensions to these concepts. The book seeks to show that, as Bull and Back point out in their introduction to another major sound studies text, *The Auditory Culture Reader*, '[t]hinking with our ears offers an opportunity to augment our critical imaginations' (2003b:2).

Methodology

The call for greater anthropological attention to the senses prompts methodological questions and concerns: how might research into the senses actually be carried out? Anthropological work on hearing demands reflection on listening and auditory engagement as key components of ethnographic fieldwork. In his introduction to *Writing Culture*, Clifford points out that: '[m]uch has been said, in criticism and praise, of the ethnographic gaze. But,' he asks, 'what of the ethnographic ear?' (1986:12). Clifford contextualizes this question by explaining that critical attention has been drawn to the inherent visualism of anthropological work. He observes that: '[t]he predominant metaphors in anthropological research have been participant observation, data collection, and cultural description, all of which presuppose a standpoint outside – looking at, objectifying, or, somewhat closer, "reading" a given reality' (ibid.:11). Clifford imagines an anthropological paradigm which no longer prefigures culture in visual terms, but which instead embraces 'a cultural poetics that is an interplay of voices' (ibid.:12). Here, 'the dominant metaphors for ethnography shift away from the observing eye and toward expressive speech' (ibid.). This shift might merit a corresponding movement away from dependence on the ethnographic eye, towards exploring the possibilities and potentials of the ethnographic ear.

Erlmann uses what he calls Clifford's 'unexpected question' as the title of his introduction to *Hearing Cultures* (2004:1). He asserts that:

> ... our quest for the ethnographic ear requires more than a metaphorical understanding of ethnography as being in need of more dialogue, more sensitized ears, or a third ear. 'Hearing Culture' suggests that it is possible to conceptualise new ways of knowing a culture and of gaining a deepened understanding of how the members of a society know each other. (ibid.:3)

Erlmann claims to use his introduction to explore some of the possible meanings of the ethnographic ear. But in fact, like Clifford, he does little to advance an understanding of how this concept might actually translate into viable empirical method. He is essentially involved in arguing for the validity of listening in anthropological work. The ethnographic ear, it seems, only serves as a general and hence somewhat vague metaphor for an auditory mode of ethnographic attention.

Discussing anthropological methodology, Cohen and Rapport (1995:12) point out that:

> Geertz's famous answer to the question, 'What does the anthropologist do? He writes', is a curiously thin description of what actually happens. Before they write, they do all those things which we gloss in the cliché of participant observation. Above all, they listen...we may not listen with sufficient care...we may listen somewhat selectively. Notwithstanding these failings, we try to listen, and to make sense of what we hear; and until we have and can show good reason for doing otherwise, we take what we hear as the expression of the speaker's consciousness.

Cohen and Rapport do not engage specifically with the idea of the ethnographic ear. They are however, strongly assertive of the importance of listening in ethnographic work, and are specific as to which sounds anthropologists prioritize in their listening. Auditory attention is, first and foremost, directed towards understanding the words spoken by those under study. For Cohen and Rapport, the ethnographic ear is primarily a verbally attuned ear.

The research on which this book is based is in part verbally eared. Interviews were conducted with doctors, patients, medical students and others. However, my ethnographic ear was also closely directed towards non-verbal (and also non-musical) sounds which occurred within the hospital and which were experienced by the people living and working there: the sounds created by the activity taking place on the wards, the sounds made by various medical technologies, the body sounds to which doctors and medical students listened when conducting auscultation and so on. Indeed, interviews were often directed towards my reaching an understanding of the meanings these sounds held for my interviewees. As Feld indicates was the case in his research among the Kaluli, learning about the way in which others hear the world involved both discussions with individuals and broader forms of 'community consultation', with auditory ethnographic attention shifting between verbal and non-verbal sounds which in turn inform one another (Feld and Brenneis 2004:487).

Pink gives careful consideration to the practice of sensory ethnography. She writes that the sensory ethnographer should 'seek routes through which to develop experienced-based, empathetic understandings of what others might be experiencing and knowing' (2009:65). In my fieldwork, the ethnographic ear that I adopted could be understood as situated and emplaced, like the ears of my interlocutors, in the hospital. I found the effort to listen through immersion in the ward environment to be essential to developing an empathetic understanding of patient experiences of hospital sounds. The fact that I was not hospitalized myself, and that therefore my listening was not influenced, for instance, by the same kind of anxiety over health issues as no doubt affected the majority of patients, is a shortcoming of the research for which I am grateful rather than regretful. In exploring auscultation, my fieldwork involved participating in classes in which students learned to listen. I attempted to develop the same skills in listening to the body sounds as they did, undertaking an apprenticeship in listening, following and reflecting on the pedagogic strategies used by the teaching doctors. This 'ears on' approach was essential to enabling me to understand how auditory knowledge was applied, reproduced and transmitted in the medical setting, and allowed me to grasp thoroughly the embodied nature of medical skill (Lachmund 1999:440).

In addition to allowing me to engage directly with the sensory intricacies of auscultation, I found that unexpected opportunities to collect data and make observations could also emerge indirectly from my apprenticeship in listening. For instance, during teaching sessions Dr Coltart would often emphasize to his students the importance of 'listening again', of going back to listen to particular heart sounds several times to be sure that we knew them and would recognize them in future. Listening again was an important teaching strategy for Dr Coltart. It was also an important methodological strategy for me. Listening to a patient with the students meant that I could reintroduce myself when I went back to listen a second time. Patients would usually recognize my face, and already associated me with listening. They knew that I was familiar with their condition, and tended to be open with me about their concerns and feelings over being in hospital. Listening again also gave me opportunities to build up relationships with individual students, as we would often visit the wards in pairs. It created conversations and initiated events that deepened and enriched my ethnography. I engage further with the methodology of the project in the conclusion, but would encourage individual researchers to specify their particular applications of the ethnographic ear in order to develop and consolidate an understanding both of the centrality to ethnographic practice of listening and its versatility as a research strategy. At the same time, it is important that the ethnographic ear does not become severed altogether from the wider sensory and embodied consciousness of the ethnographer. The concept should continue to reflect awareness that listening is embedded within, creates and sustains forms of sociality that extend far beyond auditory engagement alone.

Synopsis of chapters

Chapter 1 engages with nurses' practices of surveillance on the hospital wards, examining monitory listening and the value of sounds in focusing attention and prompting action in that setting. It introduces Foucault's discussion of panopticism and situates monitory listening as a type of acoustic surveillance that often reinforces visual surveillance. But the chapter also deepens and expands our understanding of surveillance by exploring how patients become conscious of the presence of authority through listening, and by showing the centrality of sounds to patients' experience of themselves as 'patient selves'.

Chapter 2 continues to explore patients' experiences of hospital sounds. It describes how, in the communal environment of the ward, patients are brought into often uncomfortably close proximity with one another. Sounds resist attempts to create zones of privacy as patients continually overhear their ward neighbours and are made acutely conscious that they themselves can be overheard. Hospitalization also involves the verbal disclosure of intensely private information about bodily conditions and states, while details of diagnostic information can leak out into discursive space, creating further disruptions of privacy for patients. The chapter establishes the capacity of flows of hospital sound to mark, but more often confuse and complicate bodily and spatial boundaries on the ward.

While the second chapter introduces the notion that information about the body is frequently sonically exteriorized and circulated on hospital wards, Chapter 3 focuses on the history of the acoustic exploration of the bodily interior in Western medicine. For millennia, medical practitioners have attempted to gauge the condition of the body by listening to it. Mediate auscultation or stethoscopic listening, however, substantially increased the variety of body sounds audible to the doctor and allowed sounds to be referenced to underlying physiology and pathology with far greater accuracy and specificity than had been possible with previous diagnostic listening techniques. However, the introduction of stethoscopic listening meant that doctors were obliged to hone and develop their listening skills in order to be able to detect and interpret a new 'body' of diagnostic signs. Stethoscopic listening therefore involved changes both to patients, whose bodies became acoustically intelligible, and to doctors, whose bodies became repositories of valuable specialized auditory knowledge and skill. Reflecting on the expertise required of doctors as listeners, the chapter argues that medical aurality and medical professionalization may be understood as intimately connected and as having even been co-produced.

The application of the stethoscope in a clinical situation allows for a particularly neat performance of doctorly knowledge and skill. The instrument not only mediates sounds, but through its use in auscultation also serves to structure and reinforce a particular type of doctor-patient relationship. However, Chapter 4 shows that stethoscopes are also involved in the mediation of relationships between doctors themselves and in the production and reproduction of the professional hierarchy within the hospital. It examines what might be called the 'stethoscope politics' evident at St Thomas', whereby the type of stethoscope a doctor wears, and the manner in which it is worn, can be understood as an expression of his or her relative status. Drawing on anthropological work that explores the agency of objects, the chapter highlights how many doctors depend on the stethoscope not only in order to carry out diagnostic listening, but also to articulate the nuances of their clinical persona and to reconfirm to themselves and others their identity as medical professionals.

Examining the challenges faced by medical students encountering stethoscopic listening for the first time, Chapter 5 also explores the strategies employed by teaching doctors to help students overcome these difficulties. While listening has been described as a 'technique of the body', or part of a wider 'habitus', the chapter suggests that the scale and ambition of the habitus concept makes it inappropriate as a structure through which to engage with the detail and complexity of the acquisition of a sensory skill (Mauss 1979 [1935], Bourdieu 1980). The habitus concept is also underpinned by an assumed bodily and sensory homogeneity, but, drawing on the experience of a hearing-impaired medical student, the chapter underscores the variation that in fact exists in perceptual abilities among students and illustrates the manner in which teachers are obliged to accommodate and respond to this variation. Rather than homogenizing and rendering static the medical community it describes, the chapter demonstrates that the transmission of auditory knowledge is in fact a site for the production of difference and that education in auscultation is an ongoing creative affair.

As part of learning to auscultate, students are obliged to practise listening on actual patients, particularly those who have heart sounds which teaching doctors consider to have high instructive value. These patients, and the sounds their hearts produce, frequently become the focus of numerous stethoscopic examinations and Chapter 6 considers patients' experiences of repeated auscultation. Many patients describe feeling objectified as clinical curiosities. The chapter discusses the nuances of the term 'objectification', which anthropological work on the senses has tended to position as intrinsic to vision and acts of looking. Audition and listening, on the other hand, have been imagined as creating participatory and inclusive forms of sensory engagement that do not involve objectification. By considering the notion that objectification may be brought about through auscultation as an acoustic practice, the chapter gives a reappraisal of the perceptual possibilities of audition. At the same time, the association of auscultation with acoustic objectification allows the chapter to draw out some intriguing and unexpected qualities of or potentials within the doctor-patient relationship.

The medical students with whom I studied were encouraged to listen to their own heart sounds in order to develop a sense of what normal heart sounds are like and to improve their familiarity with the cardiac cycle, a practice known as auto-auscultation. Chapter 7 describes this and also other instances of auto-auscultation in which patients listen to their own heart sounds. It goes on to describe an unusual form of auto-auscultation in which patients' heart sounds are sufficiently loud and noticeable to be audible to them without the use of a stethoscope. While the sounds made by the beating heart are usually only at the very fringes of consciousness, through auto-auscultation they become amplified and are unusually prominent in the listener's awareness of his or her own body. Auditory attention or self-exposure to the workings of one's own body is often experienced as disturbing; for those with underlying health problems, listening to their own hearts or hearing their unusually loud heart sounds can become part of an immediate experience of being unwell. The chapter shows that sound may be central not only to medical techniques of diagnosing and monitoring illness, but also to patient experiences of illness and disease.

At the time of fieldwork, auscultation was considered a valuable skill. Chapter 8, however, explores how, in the clinical environment in which my research took place, echocardiography (which uses ultrasound to produce a visual depiction of the working heart) was felt by many to be rendering auscultation obsolete. Auscultation was even said by some to be 'a dying art'. This chapter explores the 'sensory politics' behind this identified technological shift and corresponding transfer of diagnostic authority (Valente *et al.* 2011). It compares auscultation as an essentially auditory technique with echocardiography (despite its use of ultrasound) as a fundamentally visual one, whilst considering a cultural preference for visual evidence found in Western medicine. Interestingly, in some discussions over its potential demise, auscultation is identified as a technique that, unlike other diagnostic technologies, involves personal interaction between doctor and patient, fostering a relationship grounded in sympathy and empathy. The chapter argues that the fact that auscultation is an acoustic technique means it is amenable to appropriation as a symbol of sympathetic medicine, hearing having been consistently associated with inclusive, participatory engagement and with the creation of affect. The chapter therefore draws attention to the involvement of sensory politics in moral as well as pragmatic concerns, within (and by implication beyond) medical practice.

Overall, these chapters set out to reveal some of the experiential and conceptual complexity that is generated by a consideration of sound and listening in the hospital environment. They reveal some of the diversity of both professional and lay listening practices, but also point to ways in which these practices are linked. The chapters show that sound and listening have unexpected applications and implications in the medical institutions studied, so that the hospital can be understood to be saturated with sensory and specifically sonic meaning.

CHAPTER 1

Soundselves

Sound, Surveillance and Selfhood on Hospital Wards

This chapter examines the listening practices of nurses and patients on the hospital wards in which I conducted research. It considers the differing auditory perspectives that nurses and patients bring to the sounds that characterize the ward environment. The initial focus is on nurses' use of 'monitory listening', which allows them not only to check unsanctioned behaviours (although it can serve this purpose) but also to detect problems and ensure the effective management of patients on the wards. Importantly, the sounds made by medical equipment and particularly electrocardiograph machines (often known as 'heart monitors'), show that it is not only patients' actions and behaviours that are subject to aural surveillance from nurses in hospital; patients' bodies are also subject to sometimes close and protracted observation and the sounds of machines involved in techniques of bodily surveillance may feed into nurses' monitory listening. In addition, the chapter points to the use of monitory listening in the (partial) management of noise on the wards. Introducing Foucault's discussion of panopticism, it aims to convey a sense of how aural surveillance is practised in ways that often complement or interact with forms of visual surveillance.

In his work on bell ringing in the nineteenth century French countryside, Corbin (1998) indicates that surveillance may be exercised through the production of sound in addition to strategies of listening. Bells, he suggests, prompt and co-ordinate work and other activities sanctioned by those agencies with the authority to order and execute ringing. Chimes serve to reaffirm and remind those within earshot of, for instance, religious and political allegiances and duties. At the same time, they impose temporal structure and routine on the lives of those people within earshot of the bell tower. Just as people in the surrounding countryside might be observed from a belfry, they could also be reached through the sounds of the bell. Drawing on this notion from Corbin, and expanding upon Foucault by considering the potential of 'panaudicism', the chapter sets out to explore how surveillance is also articulated and exercised through the production of sounds.

Sounds on the hospital wards are not generally produced in as conscious, direct or strategic a manner as bells are rung. Through considering some patient experiences of the hospital soundscape, however, the chapter illustrates how, even when construed as unintentional by-products of medical activities and practices, the sounds of the ward can function as a kind of surveillance mechanism, indicating the presence of authority and specifying institutional rhythms and routines. For some patients, the sounds of the ward serve as a persistent reminder of their institutionalized situation, and of the fact that they are expected to remain on the wards, on bed rest or to follow treatment plans. Sounds produced by electrocardiograph machines, for instance, may reaffirm to patients that they are subject to persistent medical scrutiny. For those who are immersed in it, then, the ward soundscape can play an important role in creating and confirming a particular experience of patienthood, bringing patients to experience themselves as 'patient selves'.

Monitory listening

Foucault (1977) recognizes hospitals, like prisons, schools, army barracks and factories as disciplinary institutions. They are spaces in which power is directed towards the control and organization of people and behaviour. Hospitals involve the management of large numbers of people. Patients must, for instance, be sorted, categorized and spatially arranged according to the nature of their complaints. Their freedom to move around the hospital and interact with other patients must be restricted so as to limit contagion. They must be repeatedly checked to ensure that treatment is properly administered and followed, thus becoming subject to practices of monitoring and supervision. Although perhaps most obvious when directed in a hierarchical fashion (i.e. by staff over patients), the exercise of discipline within the contemporary hospital is often complex. Nurses and other medical professionals are themselves simultaneously both involved in and subject to monitoring, inspection and regulation. Their practice and conduct comes under frequent scrutiny. Discipline and control within the hospital is diffuse, potentially exercised by and encompassing everyone.

For Foucault visual surveillance is a key mechanism through which power is exercised within institutions such as hospitals. Introducing his ideas on surveillance he describes Jeremy Bentham's design for a prison known as the 'Panopticon' (ibid.:200–9). This well-known concept is that an observation tower is placed at the centre of a wider circle of cells. Through a set of windows, an observer positioned inside the tower is potentially able to see all the occupants of the cells at all times as the inner and outer walls of the cells are transparent, allowing light to perfuse the cells and the observer to see in. The Panopticon is intended to enable a small number of supervisors to watch over a large number of supervisees. Intervention can quickly be directed towards those whose behaviour is perceived to be deviant in any way. Although a design for a prison, the Panopticon is 'polyvalent' (ibid.:205). It enables supervisors to keep a large number of people of any kind, be they prisoners, madmen, workers, school children or importantly for the purposes of this chapter, patients, under surveillance at one time (ibid.).

In the Panopticon design the windows of the observation tower are covered by blinds or screens or are made of one way mirror glass, ensuring that an inmate cannot tell whether he is being watched or not. Thus, while the disciplinary subject 'is seen... he does not see' (ibid.:200). Conscious that he may be being observed at any time, the subject begins to monitor his own behaviour, internalizing the disciplinary gaze. He exercises surveillance upon himself, modifying his behaviour so as to conform to the rules of the institution within which he is living. The Panopticon is an especially efficient mechanism of control because the inmate becomes complicit in his own subjection.

As Gallagher points out, '[t]here is a clear consensus among Foucault scholars that his account of the Panopticon is most useful if it is understood as an ideal model for the exercise of power, rather than as a description of how specific institutions actually function' (2010:262). The Panopticon 'is a diagram of a mechanism of power reduced to its ideal form' (Foucault 1977:205). However, the Panopticon, or more broadly, panopticism has nonetheless been a useful conceptual tool in empirical research on institutions. Researchers have noted, for instance, the importance of panoptic strategies of disciplinary gazing and surveillance in schools (Gallagher 2010, Gallagher 2011, Bushnell 2003, Blackford 2004) and prisons (Reed 2004, Bart 2005). These strategies are also evident on hospital wards, and in fact Foucault writes that modern hospitals were intentionally designed to allow for the 'better observation of patients, and therefore a better calibration of their treatment' (1977:172). Ensuring their visibility was part of a deliberate strategy to enable the efficient and effective management of patients.

The hospitals in which I conducted research had a mixture of older wards built to the Nightingale Pavilion plan and more modern wards containing bays of beds with between four and eight beds to a bay. The Nightingale Pavilion plan might be considered the 'classic' hospital ward form, consisting of long, rectangular rooms with beds at regular intervals along the walls. One of the advantages of this design is that it allows all patients to be within the gaze of nurses, who are often based at stations in the centre or at the top of the ward. The arrangement allows nurses to see where care is necessary and duly administer it. Patients can be placed so that those sickest or most needing of attention are nearest the nurses' station. On the wards that consisted of bed bays, the visibility of patients to the nurses on duty was less immediate and patients could often be out of direct view of the nurses' station. However, the bed bays still allowed nurses to make quick checks of several patients at once by walking just a short distance from the station. The spatial organization of the wards, then, was designed to enable visual surveillance.

Gallagher issues a reminder that 'despite the ocularcentrism of the original blueprint, there is no reason to suppose that disciplinary surveillance must be limited to the realm of the visual' (2010:268). He cites Foucault in support of this statement: 'the procedures of power resorted to in modern societies are far too numerous and diverse and rich. It would be false to say that the principle of visibility has dominated the whole technology of power since the 19th century' (Foucault 1996:227, cited ibid.). Gallagher looks to expand our grasp of the possibilities and potentials of panopticism, and suggests that questioning its visual underpinnings might be productive in this regard. In his research on a Scottish primary school, Gallagher examines contexts in which surveillance was 'exercised through sound and hearing as much as through vision' (ibid.:262).

Acoustic surveillance was certainly noticeable on the wards, and acted as a reinforcement of or complement to visual surveillance. We see a kind of 'panauralism' being applied alongside the visual gazing associated with panopticism (ibid.:268). This aural surveillance was perhaps most obvious in the monitory listening practised by nurses. As described in more detail below, this listening was sometimes directed towards the detection of any inappropriate or unacceptable behaviour. More often, though, it was focused on sounds that indicated that a patient required attention or that there was a problem. For instance, on one occasion I was speaking to a nurse when she held up a finger to interrupt me and cocked her head to one side. She had noticed a particular sound and was now listening carefully. She then got up and walked to the bedside of a patient who was breathing with the assistance of an oxygen mask. Having made an adjustment to the mask she came back to the station. It seemed that the mask had slipped or been knocked, meaning that oxygen was escaping. The nurse had noticed that the sound it had been making was 'not right', and this had prompted her to intervene. On another occasion I was conducting an interview when a patient in a nearby bed who was eating began to cough and appeared to be choking. The noise caught the attention of a nurse working perhaps fifteen metres away across the ward. She stopped what she was doing and came to help. When, a few minutes later, she left the bedside, the patient was calm and sat more upright than before, having been propped up with pillows. On the ward, then, monitory listening played an important part in attracting and focusing visual attention and prompting action. While Foucault considers the panopticon design to allow supervisors to see and if necessary quickly intervene in inmate behaviour, for nurses sounds play an important role in their supervision of patient populations.

It was possible for nurses to continue their monitory listening whilst engaged in other tasks that might occupy their visual attention. As Gallagher points out, '[w]hereas the human eyes are directional, human ears have greater capacity to capture information from all around' (2011:51). Nurses can keep an ear out for signals within the ward soundscape whilst also concerning themselves with matters closer to hand. Perhaps the best analogy is with a parent listening to a baby monitor. He or she can carry on with a visually and partly acoustically absorbing activity, also attending but not responding to sounds of rest, sleep, low volume speech or benign movement relayed by the system, yet being able to respond quickly to unacceptably loud noise or to sounds that might indicate distress or constitute an appeal for help.

The monitory listening practised by nurses might seem to bear similarities to stethoscopic listening: they are trying to listen to the ward as if it were a body, making judgments as to which sounds are normal and which abnormal, diagnosing problems affecting patients. But stethoscopic listening, I would argue, differs in that it is a particularly concentrated form of listening that involves focusing one's full attention on one sound at a time to the exclusion of others. It is what Truax refers to as a form of 'listening-in-search' (2001:22). Monitory listening is more a form of what he calls 'listening-in-readiness', where 'the attention is in readiness to receive significant information, but where the focus of one's attention is probably directed elsewhere' (ibid.). He suggests that this particular mode of auditory awareness usually depends on a set of associations that are built up over time so that familiar noises are identified and evaluated through relatively low-level processing in the brain. The listener is able to judge subtle differences of quality in these familiar sounds, so that, for instance, a nurse might notice a cough indicating choking even against a background of other sounds.

Some medical technologies are designed to produce signals that feed into the monitory listening practised by nurses. The sounds of electrocardiograph (also known as ECG or EKG) machines were a distinctive feature of cardiothoracic wards in particular. These machines are themselves concerned with the surveillance and monitoring of the patient body, specifically the electrical activity of the heart. The most important information they produce is displayed numerically and graphically on a monitor, but they can also be set to emit audible tones that essentially prompt inspection of this data. For instance, the machine might be programmed to sound at the point of systole, which is when the ventricles of the heart contract. The frequency and pattern of the beep then gives information as to the rate and rhythm of the heartbeat. The electrocardiograph machines at St Thomas' could also be set to give a tone if the heart rate exceeded or dropped below a particular number of beats per minute, or to produce a fault tone if patients became detached from the leads connecting them to the machine. This signal could be heard at some distance from the bedside of the patient being monitored, allowing nurses to carry out tasks nearby whilst keeping the tones at the periphery of their attention, responding if necessary. Similarly, some drips were administered to patients by being attached to small units called 'infusion pumps' that could be used to regulate the flow of liquid; these machines emitted programming tones when the intended rate was being set. However, they also produced a fault tone when there were problems with the pumps, or when drips required replacement or refilling. On hearing the tone, nurses would generally respond and take steps to address the issue being signalled.

Patients were conscious that there were listening ears around them and, as explored in detail in the following chapter, were troubled by the loss of privacy their audibility on the wards entailed. They were aware of a kind of acoustic exposure that made it difficult for them to create or guard a sense of privacy. But knowing that both they and the equipment to which they were attached could be heard as well as seen was also potentially reassuring. They knew that if they were to show a sign of distress, call or cry out, or if there were to be a problem with a machine, there was a good chance that a nurse would notice and come to help. Surveillance, then, is not necessarily only restrictive or controlling in its implications. Here, it potentially empowers patients, enabling them to lay claim to the attention and expertise of the nurses.

Discontinuous monitoring

Another piece of equipment that fed into the monitory listening practised by nurses was what was variously referred to as a 'call', 'help' or 'assistance' button. At St Thomas', this was found on a small control panel attached by a cable to the wall at the head of the bed. The panel also had buttons that could be used to change the height of the bed and allow the incline of its top half to be altered. Importantly, the 'call' button served as a guarantee of a patient's audibility and visibility where panopticism and panauralism might otherwise fail or be incomplete. Pressing the button produced a tone and/or activated a light at the nurses' station, making the patient both heard and seen, provided of course that the station was manned.

Sometimes nurses would be too busy or engrossed in an urgent task to respond to a call for help or a fault tone from a machine, and would ignore it. If numerous claims were being made on their attention it was necessary for them to make decisions as to which to prioritize. But conditions on the ward could also present barriers to effective listening. Above I suggested that monitory listening could be considered a form of 'listening-in-readiness'. Truax notes, however, that this kind of listening 'requires a favourable environmental situation for it to be effective...a minimum signal-to-noise ratio is required so that the desired signal may be separated from any competing noise' (2001:23). Excessive noise is an acoustic barrier to listening-in-readiness, akin to a pall of smoke obscuring a person's view. The ward was generally a busy sonic environment and machine tones were almost constantly in competition with one another and with sounds from, for instance, the telephone at the nurses' station, the notifier tones produced by the pagers worn by doctors and other hospital staff, and other tones whose origin, despite careful observation and questioning, I was unable to determine. This was in addition to all the sounds produced by other activities taking place on the ward. It is perhaps not surprising that nurses sometimes excused their not having responded to a call or an alarm sound because they simply had not heard it.

No doubt some nurses were less perceptive of the sounds around them than others. I was told that no formal training was given in monitory listening. Levels of skill in this mode of auditory attention were therefore likely to vary, just as skill, knowledge and experience in other nursing tasks no doubt vary to an extent even among those of the same professional grade. At the same time, responsiveness to sounds would depend on individual nurses' levels of energy, rigour and conscientiousness. These would never be perfectly consistent, meaning that auditory surveillance would never be absolutely constant.

Patients were aware that auditory surveillance was 'discontinuous', and knew that the nature of the acoustic environment on the ward meant that if they needed a nurse's attention they would sometimes have to make a conscious effort to get it (Gallagher 2010:266). This was shown, for instance, on one occasion when I observed a patient who was anxious about an alarm tone issuing from his infusion pump. He had noticed a nurse walk past (she had in fact been answering a help call from another patient) without attending to it. 'Why doesn't this machine like me?' he asked, loudly, as she walked back past him a few minutes later. She stopped and addressed the problem. In a similar case, another patient was irritated by the fault tone the ECG equipment to which he was attached was making. After several minutes of the tone sounding he asked a passing nurse if she could stop it.

At times, then, patients could also become involved in forms of monitory listening. They were particularly alert to the sounds made by the machines to which they were attached. But they also listened to sounds from other patients. On two occasions that I observed, patients who were very ill called out, but only loudly enough to be heard by those in beds next to them or very nearby. These ward neighbours then relayed the calls more loudly to the nurses to make sure that they were aware there was a problem. In a sense, patients were monitoring the monitory listening of the nurses. They were sensitive to its weaknesses, and knew that amplification was at times necessary to ensure important messages were heard and followed by a proper response.

Sometimes, though, nurses felt that particular patients were unnecessarily demanding, repeatedly calling for help or sounding the assistance button and then asking them to do the smallest tasks of which the patients themselves might be easily capable, like filling a glass of water or rearranging a sheet. Nurses would complain to one another that these patients were 'bossy', treated the hospital as if it was a hotel or acted as if the nurses were their servants. In these situations, 'not hearing' could become a potential excuse for a deliberate decision not to respond as much as an explanation for accidental neglect. Monitory listening created potential for acts of resistance, a response to patients' more obvious attempts to exercise power over their nurse supervisors.

Quiet wards?

In his ethnographic research on a Scottish primary school, Gallagher was impressed by teachers' intense focus on maintaining quiet in the classroom (2010:268). Noise levels, he observed, were constantly subject to surveillance. Noise control was partly maintained through sight, for instance by teachers looking to see who might be making noise. But hearing was also used, so that teachers listened out for unsanctioned behaviours as well. At the same time, they would verbally remind pupils that their exchanges and activities could be heard. Children were thus made to 'hear that they could always be heard' (Gallagher 2011:51). While teachers might not notice some unregulated noise, pupils were made conscious of their almost permanent potential audibility.

Schwartz (2012) indicates that quiet has for millennia been considered the best sonic environment in which to heal the sick. The therapeutic value of quiet is described in Egyptian, Greco-Roman, Jewish and Islamic medical traditions and has been incorporated into modern Euro-American notions of the optimum environment for treatment and recovery (ibid.:273–4). Florence Nightingale, an influential figure in the development of modern nursing (who had a nursing school at St Thomas' and now has a ward named after her there), maintained that quiet was vital to the wellbeing of patients (ibid.:274–7). Schwartz also notes that some hospitals and sanatoria, including Quaker-run asylums, imposed 'therapeutic quietudes' on patients, just as 'punitive-penitent quietudes' had been imposed on those imprisoned under the Silent System (ibid.:274).

Nurses to whom I spoke during fieldwork considered silence undesirable. Those I asked said that the ideal ward soundscape was quiet. Loud noise tended to indicate dramatic events and emergencies requiring urgent action and intervention. It suggested a lack of control over the ward and its patients. Silence, which I took to refer here not to a complete absence of sounds, but to a subdued sonic environment or one characterized by an absence of people, they equated with death. A relatively low-level murmur or hum of activity was best. As one nurse explained:

> I certainly prefer to hear everyday sounds like snoring, sometimes breathing, chatting with visitors, that kind of thing... Big shouts or a hubbub spells an emergency, danger. That's scary and gets the adrenaline going. Silence, though, that's the worst. If there's silence you know it's too late. That's when it's over.

Here we see an additional level of monitory listening practised by nurses, a generalized sensitivity to the character of the ward soundscape as a whole.

My patient interlocutors often experienced the wards as being disturbingly noisy. There is a clear tension produced by the fact that quiet is culturally endorsed as the most appropriate environment for convalescence, while the hospital ward is a communal space where (increasingly technologically intense) medical work takes place. Yet noise levels on the ward were subject to some regulation. When unacceptably loud noise or disruption which did not have immediate medical import occurred, nurses would take steps to intervene, requesting for instance, that patients (and/or visitors) who were talking particularly loudly be quieter out of consideration for others. Patients were also allowed to see as well as hear that they could be heard: nurses were in relative proximity and would meet noisy interactions between patients with raised eyebrows, frowns and other gentle rebukes. Patients who persistently made unacceptably loud (either voluntary or involuntary) vocalizations would where possible be moved to a side ward where they would create less of a disturbance. This was the case, for instance, with a lady I encountered during my research who was particularly hostile and who frequently made loud, offensive remarks to the medical staff and to other patients.

Although efforts were made to prevent excessive noise on the wards during the day, the focus on maintaining at least a degree of quiet became most noticeable at night. On the cardiothoracic wards at St Thomas', as the lights were dimmed at around 9.30 there was a corresponding effort to lower sound levels. This partly manifested itself in aural self-surveillance by the nurses. They often spoke in gentler tones to one another and to patients than they had during the day, implying that patients should do the same and monitor their own noise making. I noticed that they would often, for instance, lift privacy curtains slightly as they pulled them so that the hooks did not scrape too loudly along the rails, something they might not have done during the day. In low voices they would ask patients having loud conversations to speak quietly. Shortly after completing my fieldwork I spent a night in hospital myself following a septoplasty (an operation to straighten a deviated nasal septum). A man in an adjacent bed-bay was very agitated; he repeatedly shouted and cried out during the night, waking other patients and preventing them from sleeping. Eventually he was given a sedative, which may well have been beneficial to him but also had the effect of quickly restoring a normal night-time noise level to the ward. I did not see this happen during fieldwork, but I suspect that patients were sometimes medicated in order to ensure calm on wards.

Given their high degree of exposure to the sounds of the ward and often their inability to escape it, many patients themselves acted to ensure that a degree of acoustic discipline was maintained. During the night I spent in hospital patients had complained numerous times to the nurses on duty that the disturbance the man was creating was unacceptable. On several occasions during fieldwork I also saw patients asking other patients and their visitors to talk more quietly, and I even observed patients asking nurses to be quieter in their chatting and laughter at the nurses' station. As Gallagher reminds us, the roles of surveyor and surveyed are available to all (2010:266). Ultimately, surveillance is all-encompassing. It is a system which entraps everyone.

Auditory self-surveillance was also noticeable on the wards. Most patients were careful to monitor the noise they made out of consideration for the other patients. In order to protect their own dignity they also took pains to restrict potentially embarrassing sounds (of bodily functions, for example) in the communal space of the wards. Patients here may be seen to be regulating their own behaviour, exercising control themselves, independently and spontaneously, in ways that reinforce the apparent institutional aim of producing (reasonably) quiet spaces occupied by (reasonably) quiet persons.

I have argued here that nurses made an effort to maintain some degree of quiet, at least at night. Yet, as indicated above, patients were often disturbed by noise. This apparent contradiction resolves itself when we consider the different acoustic perspectives that patients and nurses respectively bring to the ward. It is easy to see, for instance, that the persistent beeping sound produced by an electrocardiograph might be loud and irritating, if not for the patient being monitored, then for his or her ward neighbours. For a nurse, however, this same signal might carry important information, and its steady repetitions might be reassuring to him or her as an indicator of a patient's stable condition. At the same time, a patient who is a 'captive audience' to the ward soundscape for twenty-four hours a day is perhaps likely to be more irritated by its monotonous and repetitive or sudden and alarming sounds than a nurse who is there for perhaps ten hours at a time, and who frequently moves around the ward (Kittay 2008). These differences of perspective continue: a patient's priority is often rest and recuperation, whilst a nurse's is the completion of tasks; patients are likely to be ill and weak, more sensitive to noise and its disruptive effect on their rest, while nurses are likely to be more robust and will be largely unaffected by any disturbing sonic presences. Despite efforts to control noise levels, a ward can easily be noisy and quiet at the same time depending on the acoustic perspective, or earpoint of the listener.

Panaudicism

Thus far we have considered the monitory listening practised by nurses in relation to the management of patients and their conditions. While I was researching at the Edinburgh Royal Infirmary, I met a man named Anthony who was a particularly rebellious patient. Anthony's account of his hospital experience drew my attention to the manner in which sound making on the part of nurses and listening practices on the part of patients might also be bound up with the exercise of surveillance within the hospital.

Anthony was a man of thirty-two who had been given six weeks bed-rest in order to allow a smashed elbow and a fractured pelvis to heal. This meant he was unable to get off his bed except to wheelchair himself to the toilet and to his daily physiotherapy sessions. He was, then, largely confined to the ward. Although recovering from serious injury, Anthony proudly informed me that he was known as the ward troublemaker. He had twice been caught smoking and once got drunk on vodka that a friend had smuggled in disguised as mineral water. He took great pleasure in recounting how he had succeeded in buying hash from one of the cleaners. Anthony expressed a willingness to exchange information for pornographic magazines. Three *Fiestas* and a couple of *Knaves* later he agreed to be interviewed. His mischievous activities, he said, had only been possible since being transferred from the main ward to a small side ward where his was the only bed. In the main ward he had been aware of being constantly watched by the nurses. 'They were all over the bloody place,' he said. 'Always saying "What do you think you're doing?" and "Where do you think you're going?" It was claustrophobic if you know what I mean.' While the use of visual and possible aural surveillance is apparent here, Anthony told me that it was most often the sounds of the nurses that reminded him of his being under observation. During the day their voices and activity, footsteps and even the swish of their clothing meant he was unable to forget that authority was not far away. Rolling a cigarette on the windowsill one day, he had thought he heard a nurse approaching. Panicking, he pushed his papers and tobacco out of the window. It was a false alarm.

Foucault suggests that the Panopticon prison design represents a highly efficient mechanism for discipline and control because, conscious that their every move might be being observed, inmates internalize the disciplinary gaze and come to monitor their own behaviour. This minimizes the need for the supervisors to act and intervene. Power is exercised 'spontaneously', and interestingly, Foucault remarks, 'without noise' (1977:206). His implication is that control may be exercised swiftly and with precision. Noise here seems to indicate unnecessary action and fuss. However, while Foucault uses an acoustic term to indicate a loss of efficiency in the exercise of power, Anthony clearly experiences sound as an auditory complement to surveillance, making it more pervasive and effective. Just as the click of a camera asserts that a picture has been taken, or the whirr of a closed circuit TV camera informs a person that his movements are being watched, the sound of nurses suggested to him that he was under their attentive eyes. As well as hearing that he could be heard, Anthony heard that he could be seen. Sounds here embody the presence of authority, reinforcing the system of surveillance. Indeed, the sounds of authority pervade a space that the disciplinary gaze cannot reach: Anthony heard the sound at a moment when he was deliberately concealing his actions from view.

Bull and Back point out that Bentham's Panopticon was not only an apparatus for the visual exercise of power, but was also 'a listening prison in which, through a series of tubes, the inmates could be heard at all times' (2003b:5). Markus (1993) and Johnston (2000) also indicate that Bentham's original design for the Panopticon included listening tubes to complement and extend visual surveillance. Above, we have seen techniques of listening being used to extend the scope of panoptic possibility. But the situation described by Anthony also lends a new dimension to the acoustics of power. Control is not effected through the possibility of being heard by an omnipresent authoritarian presence, but in hearing an authoritarian presence. We see a similar notion emerging in Sartre's *Being and Nothingness*, where the author imagines himself looking through a keyhole, spying on a scene inside a room. He knows his spying is an illicit act and so the sound of an approaching footstep is an immediate reproach. It suggests to him that he has been seen by another person: '[h]ere I am bent over the keyhole; suddenly I hear a footstep. I shudder as a wave of shame sweeps over me. Somebody has seen me. I straighten up. My eyes run over the deserted corridor' ([1943] 2002:277). The sound creates the sense of being watched, and seems to make other people present all around. '[E]ach creak', Sartre writes, 'announces to me a look', because 'I am already in the state of being-looked-at' (ibid.). Interestingly, as in Anthony's case, '[i]t was a false alarm' (ibid.). Sound creates a kind of spectre, a 'sinister resonance'; the ghostly present absence or absent presence of authority (Toop 2010).

The situations described by Anthony and Sartre illustrate the possibility not of panauralism, but of what, to rework the panopticon term from Foucault, might be described as panaudicism. This operates through the infiltration of sounds that signify authoritarian presences into the patient's awareness. The inmate, as well as the supervisor's ear, thus becomes an important channel of power, a sensory avenue through which power acts. The inmate becomes the bearer of a receptive ear/eye of power, as well as the object of an ear/eye of power. Of course, it is probable that, as a rebellious patient, Anthony was the focus of more disciplinary attention than would be employed with most other patients. Nonetheless, I feel his experience gives important indications for developing our understanding of the possibilities of the involvement of sound in surveillance. Of course, there is a flipside to the situation described by Anthony. He found that the auditory presence of authority was oppressive. But for some other patients, hearing the sound of nurses, knowing that they were close (and thus hearing that they themselves could be heard and seen) could be reassuring. They knew that if they were to call or cry out a nurse would notice and come to help. Here, the reassuring, as much as the oppressive presence of authority also articulates itself sonically.

Soundselves

Above I cited Corbin's work on village bells in the nineteenth century French countryside. One of the points he makes is that the sounding of bells was an expression of dominance over the space in which those bells could be heard. Corbin goes on to point out that '[b]ells did not only serve as auditory markers. They also played a part... in the marking that served to constitute a territory, and that was indissociable from the notion of surveillance' (1998:210). Here Corbin echoes Attali's assertion that sound is a tool for the demarcation of space and as such plays a fundamental role in the claiming and specification of territory (Attali 1985:6). But he also offers up the notion that surveillance may be exercised through the production of sound. Sounding bells denote the presence, dominance and authority of those who order them rung and/or who carry out the ringing. At the same time they act as prompts or summonses for activities such as work, religious observances, community meetings and so on. Sounding bells serve to structure the behaviour of those within earshot. A kind of overseeing-through-sound takes place. In institutions such as schools and prisons, this type of surveillance through sound-making is apparent when bells, claxons and other sonic devices are used to impose particular rhythms on institutional life, to prompt activities, co-ordinate the movement of persons and so on.

Following Corbin, the sounds of medical work that dominate the wards might be understood both to demarcate those spaces as a medical territory and to demarcate the patients within them as subject to medical authority. This is not necessarily accomplished deliberately through the actions of a particular individual or group. Rather, it is a consequence of the medical purpose of hospital wards and of the practices that take place within them. Anthony's account of his experience of being in hospital is an instance of how, as Corbin suggests, surveillance may be exercised through the production of sound. However, in his case this did not take place in a way that was obviously planned or co-ordinated as might be suggested by the carefully timed and deliberate ringing of a bell. Instead, it was patterns of noise that might be understood as by-products of the activities and practices taking place on the ward that provoked a consciousness of the presence of the authority.

Patients to whom I spoke also indicated that the sounds of the hospital served to impose routines, to create and reinforce the pattern of institutional life. Above I referred to nurses' attempts to create a night-time ward environment by dimming the lights and trying to ensure a greater degree of quiet than had been possible during the day. But both patients and nurses also made reference to a 'dawn chorus' on the ward. This generally began at around 6.00, and gradually intensified as patients woke and stirred, made trips to the toilets, spoke to one another and to the nurses and so on. Nurses, too, would be active during this period, checking on patients as they woke. The nurses did not seem to make efforts to control or mute the 'dawn chorus', but allowed it to perform the function of a slow-acting alarm clock. Their charges would, after all, generally need to be woken for breakfast and/or prepared for the morning ward round. Patients also came to recognize other phases and events within the institutional day by the sounds that accompanied them. They could tell when meals or medicines were about to arrive by noticing the sound of the trolley, often some time before it became visible to them. Commenting on the sounds in the male respiratory ward at the Edinburgh Royal Infirmary, a patient named Hugh told me: 'You can tell what's going on, you know. You can hear that they're getting dinner ready, or that the medicine trolley's coming round, and you can set your watch when you hear the nurses changing shift.' Forcing themselves on patients' awareness, sounds played a role in habituating them to the pattern of institutional life, readying them for the sequence of activities there. Sounds served to entrain patients into particular habits, moulding them into patterns of behaviour. It is partly by listening to, or being exposed to its sounds that the routine of the hospital is internalized by patients.

This chapter opened by referring to Foucault's discussion of the Panopticon. Foucault understands the purpose of this architectural design as being to allow the exercise of power over inmates. Power may be directed towards punishing criminals, increasing the productivity and self-application of workers or schoolchildren, instilling discipline in soldiers and so on. In part, then, power is directed with the aim of producing 'docile' bodies, bodies that are trained, responsive and obedient (1977:135–69). In the accounts described above, sound making may also be understood to be involved in producing docile patient bodies, specifically patients who are obedient and habituated to the routines of hospital life. However, Foucault holds that while the exercise of power can serve to control people, it also serves to nurture and mould them, shaping their capacities as individuals. So while power produces subjects, it also produces subjectivity. Foucault calls this ambivalent process 'subjectivation'. As well as indicating ways in which sound and listening might play a part in the production of disciplined patient bodies, this chapter also illustrates how the sounds of the hospital are involved in the processes through which people are shaped, and shape themselves, into patient selves.

Hospital ward soundscapes are immediately and distinctly different from those associated with other domestic, public and even institutional spaces. The sounds of the activity and work of care, of medical equipment, of sick people, define the ward as a medical space. As Priscilla, a patient at the Edinburgh Royal Infirmary who referred to herself as 'one of the bladder ladies', remarked: 'With all the coughing and the noise and buzzing, where else could I be but in hospital?' James, a patient in the dermatology unit at the Infirmary, expressed the same idea: 'Sometimes when I've just woken up I lie there and think "I'd like to go for a nice walk", but hearing everything going on in the ward chases that idea away because I realize "Oh no, of course I can't, I'm sick aren't I?"' The soundscape forces James to recognize that he is in hospital. It reaffirms his patienthood. In fact, though, it does more than simply state the fact of his being institutionalized. James implies that the hospital soundscape references a particular set of restrictions. He can't, realistically, just get up, leave the ward and go for a walk. He knows it is preferred that he should stay in or near his bed, rest and receive treatment. At the very least, in order to go for a walk, he would have to negotiate permission to leave with nurses and doctors or discharge himself. The soundscape he hears, then, indexes a particular experience of patienthood, one characterized by the necessity of acting in accordance with institutional rules and protocols.

As suggested earlier in the chapter, the persistent tones of ECG machines were a noticeable feature of wards designated to cardiological medicine in particular. One patient described them as being 'the heartbeat of the ward', a sonic leitmotif of life there. Among patients to whom I spoke there was a consensus that the near-constant pulsing of the electrocardiograph was irritating. The sound was high-pitched, persistent and rarely out of earshot. 'Sometimes it makes me want to scream,' said one lady to whom I spoke. 'Can't they turn the wretched thing off from time to time?' asked the person in the adjacent bed. It seemed not. Indeed, during fieldwork I spoke to both doctors and nurses who said that they did not know how to turn the volume of the ECG unit off or down. 'When I lie there and listen to those bleeps and blinks I feel as though I were a lab-rat, something in a laboratory, you know,' remarked Carrie from the Female Cardiology Unit at the Edinburgh Royal Infirmary. 'It's very strange when even in the night all these machines are bleeping away,' said Brian who was recovering from a stroke. 'They never stop, and you think to yourself "What kind of place am I in?"' As was the case with James, for these patients the sounds of the ward, and especially the ECG, constitute something more than just an annoyance. They become symbols of a particular kind of hospitalization, one in which they are made subject to persistent medical monitoring and surveillance.

One of the patients to whom I spoke at St Thomas' had observed that the nurses were almost continually going to and fro in order to carry out observations on patients. On his particular ward this involved them taking and noting each person's blood pressure and temperature at regular intervals. Taking blood pressure often involves the inflation of a cuff around the patient's upper arm, constricting the flow of blood. This cuff is inflated either by hand, using a small plastic pump, or automatically if the blood pressure is being taken by machine. The hand pump makes a vigorous 'sshhhh' noise each time it is compressed by the nurse, while the machine emits a steady whirring. In both cases the cuff makes a sighing sound when the air inside it is eventually released. The patient to whom I spoke said he disliked the strong feeling of constriction in the arm that the cuff produced. He likened the sigh of the escaping air to his own sighs of relief when each of his observations was over. At the same time, he explained that the sounds made around him as nurses carried out their work reminded him that, in this environment, observation and other monitoring practices were virtually continuous and unavoidable. Hearing them, he knew that he would be due for his observations again soon and at regular intervals for his entire hospital stay. Sounds for him became symbols of a patient experience dominated by medical surveillance and the obligation to make oneself available to it.

Chuengsatiansup (1999) describes how, for a group known as the Kui who live in Northeast Thailand, the loud harsh sounds of, for instance, motorbikes, machinery, carousing drunkards and rowing neighbours increasingly pervade the soundscapes of their rural villages. For the Kui, these sounds have come to symbolize the incoming forces of modernity which, they fear, will ultimately bring about the destruction of their traditional way of life. Chuengsatiansup indicates that these sounds have become closely associated with a form of illness that affects Kui women in particular. He argues that the effects of being startled by the harsh, often sudden sounds, combined with deep seated anxiety provoked by the instability and uncertainty they represent, are locally interpreted as generating an illness whose symptoms include sleeplessness, shortness of breath, feeling frightened, loss of appetite and chronic fatigue. In a related way, Sullivan (1986) explores sonic symbolism among the peoples of the highlands and Eastern Montana of the Andes. He describes how there, the screeching of industrial machinery is imagined to be the cries of a monstrous being named *Pishtaco*, who screams as he sucks out the body fat of Indians in order to lubricate car and aeroplane engines, boat motors and mining equipment. His scream is the sound of the invading industrial society and its machinery, which displaces, enslaves and ultimately destroys indigenous communities.

Both these analyses suggest that background sounds are expressive of wider social processes. I would not seek to claim that the hospital soundscape represents a cultural symbol of the same scale as the harrowing examples given by Chuengsatiansup and Sullivan. However, the notion that important meanings may be simultaneously disguised and announced in the background sounds of place, space or social setting is useful here. For patients, the hospital soundscape both symbolizes and constitutes the sonic embodiment of a particular set of institutional practices. It can be understood to indicate the presence and vigilance of nursing staff, announce and embody phases of the institutional day and articulate the persistent and pervasive application of medical surveillance. It is, partly at least, through these sounds that listening patients come to recognize and live out their hospitalized situation, their position as institutionalized 'selves'. In some patients, then, we see the emergence of a sonically ordered sense of self, a 'selfhood' shaped by the acoustic dimension.

CHAPTER 2

Broadcasting the Body

The Private Made Public in Hospital Soundscapes

We have seen that ward soundscapes are characterized by the activity and work of care: the conversations and footsteps of nurses, the rattling of medicine trolleys, the rasp of privacy curtains being drawn around beds, telephones ringing, machines beeping and so on. Overlapping and interweaving with these noises are sounds produced by the patients themselves: talking and moving around, but sometimes also coughing, sobbing, vomiting, emitting cries of pain or delirium. With their movement often severely restricted, many patients I observed found themselves to be a captive audience to the sounds that were constantly being broadcast across the ward. Patients not accustomed to hospital visits were often deeply affected by the soundscape that surrounded them there. Many expressed surprise and, more often than not, distaste at the kinds of sounds to which they were exposed, and at the volume, intensity and frequency of disturbance.

Not all patients were sensitive to the soundscape of the ward. Some longer-term patients had grown accustomed to its acoustic profile in the way 'the sound of a waterfall soon becomes an unheard sound to those who live near it' (Kesey 1973:75). Existing research suggests that people can become habituated to certain recurrent sounds and sometimes cease to notice them altogether (Medical Research Council 1997:36). As part of his sound art project on the Harefield Transplant Hospital, Wynne (2007) interviewed a patient (in fact a qualified doctor herself) who explained that she eventually became somewhat less sensitive to what she had at first experienced as the very loud and disturbing sounds of the ward in which she was staying. She also described a (not entirely successful) strategy of trying to imagine the intrusive tones and alarms of medical technologies as the bleating of Greek sheep and goats up a mountainside. This technique of re-imagining potentially bothersome sounds as elements of soundscapes with more pleasant associations is also well illustrated by Bachelard ([1958] 1994:28–9). He details a process of trying to reinvent the noises of the city that envelop his Paris bedroom as an ocean soundscape. None of my patient interlocutors, however, described using this kind of imaginative reworking of the soundscape as a coping mechanism, and although they would make efforts to block out the sounds around them, toleration of the sounds of the wards was, in the main, partial and limited.

Suzanne Cusick (2006, 2008, 2013) describes the use of sound and music in the detention camps of the global war on terror. Inmates relate their experiences of a kind of 'acoustic dystopia' in which loud music is used strategically to disorientate, demoralize and even debilitate (2013:285). The present chapter is concerned with a different 'sonics of suffering' from a different kind of institution (Gunaratnam 2009:3). But as in the context studied by Cusick, sound becomes notable as an agent or vector of discomfort and anxiety, its dynamics even presenting a challenge to the preservation of normal subjectivity.

On entering hospital, patients are no longer able to exercise control over the physical and social proximity or distance they maintain in relation to others. In public hospitals in particular, patients are often obliged to spend each phase of their daily existence (sleeping, eating and so on) in the company of relative strangers (both patients and staff) sharing a managed communal space. In both of the institutions in which I conducted research, patients remarked that upon being admitted to hospital 'the first thing you lose is your privacy, the second is your dignity and the third is your sanity'. Their use of this exact phrase made me think that it had been passed between patients and hospitals across the country and could perhaps be aligned with a distinct patient culture.

It is certainly easy to see that for a person in hospital privacy is difficult to preserve. He or she must share space with others, being almost constantly under the gaze and within earshot of other patients and of medical staff. For many of the patients to whom I spoke, sounds played a key role in the loss of privacy that they identified. Many found they were unable to escape the sonic detail of the suffering of their ward neighbours. Sounds would infiltrate and pervade both their immediate physical environment and what they tended to describe as their 'mental space'. At the same time, most patients were acutely conscious that they themselves could be overheard by those nearby.

Whilst in hospital, patients become the objects or recipients of a range of diagnostic, management and treatment practices which, like the inhabitation of shared space, often necessitate the invasion or compromise of privacy. A patient might have to undergo examinations or procedures that involve physical exposure and intrusion. He or she might depend on staff for intimate bodily care. At the same time, within the clinical environment, bodies are scrutinized: their surfaces, recesses, structures, tissues, fluids and processes are made subject to inspection, analysis and discussion. For my patient interlocutors, sounds were often involved in these processes of 'opening out' the body. Medical technologies conveyed sonically coded information about bodily events not only to medical professionals but also to the patients themselves and beyond, across the ward. Most patients found that they were rendered undiscriminating and inexpert listeners amidst the audible interactions of specialists and their machines.

Diagnosis and treatment also often entailed discussion, meaning that patient bodies were articulated but also distributed and dispersed through sound in the form of verbal exchanges. The previous chapter considered how hospital soundscapes make audible a field of power relations, manifested through surveillance. In this chapter power relations become apparent in the professional control of knowledge about and discourse on a patient's condition and the public disclosure of intensely private information. Details of illnesses and treatment processes were acquired, held and circulated by medical professionals. In the main, discussions about patients were confined to areas out of earshot of patients. A fairly strict segregation of discourse, a managed zoning of auditory space prevailed. Occasionally, however, medical discourse was inappropriately overheard, meaning that intensely private details about patients' bodies were allowed to enter more public zones of acoustic and discursive space. Within hospital, then, sound was experienced as exteriorizing or broadcasting information about the inner recesses of the body, crossing and confusing boundaries between inner and outer, self and other. The agency of sound to disturb, dissolve and reconfigure the boundaries of private and public space became strongly apparent.

Over-hearing

The terms 'public' and 'private' have a particularly strong resonance in relation to hospitals in the UK, where, of course, they also reference and contrast publicly and privately funded institutions. Typically better resourced than public ones, private hospitals tend to differ in terms of design. Where public hospitals like those in which I conducted research generally have large, open wards, private hospitals tend to have smaller, even individual rooms. There is a less public performance of the illness role and less exposure to the presence of other patients. Unlike many public hospitals (including both the Edinburgh Royal Infirmary and St Thomas'), private hospitals are rarely used in the teaching of medical students and so patients are unlikely to become involved in the public arena which tuition sessions represent (Sinclair 1997).

That illness in a private hospital is a comparatively private experience would doubtless be reflected in the soundscapes of these clinics.

In the communal environment of public hospital wards, certain gestures are made towards securing or preserving a vestige of visual privacy for patients. For instance, curtains are often pulled around the beds of patients undergoing examinations and procedures or receiving care. Even if all other patients on the ward are well aware of what is taking place behind it, the privacy curtain ensures they are spared the visual details. The curtain also functions as a sign that advises or even warns the onlooker: 'you should turn away' or 'for your own good, you should try not to register what is happening behind here'; after all, curtains are pulled around the beds of patients who are dying or have recently died. The privacy curtain alerts those who see it to redirect their attention, and performs a kind of theatre of consideration for individual privacy. But sound is no respecter of the privacy curtain. Sounds move under, over and through these screens. They escape the temporary area of visually 'private' space the curtain constructs, seeping or radiating out into the ward and the auditory space of others. For occupants of the ward, it is made acoustically apparent that 'each phase of the member's daily activity is carried on in the immediate company of a large batch of others' (Goffman 1968:17).

Sometimes, the sounds coming through the curtain could be harrowing for patients. One lady I spoke to grimaced as she described the whimpering which had come from behind the screen as her neighbour used a bedpan for the first time since undergoing a bowel operation. Another had had to endure prolonged cries of agony from nearby as a man underwent an unpleasant procedure hidden from view. She looked exhausted and upset as she related what had clearly been an ordeal for both of them. A man named Gordon, who had recently been discharged, described how during his stay in hospital his ward neighbour had suffered a heart attack late at night. Nursing staff had been quick to help and had pulled the privacy curtains around all the beds. A resuscitation team had been called and Gordon had been obliged to listen to the dramatic sounds of their attempts to save the man's life. Eventually he had heard them agree that their efforts had failed and after the necessary preparations had been made he heard the body wheeled away. 'I was shattered for days by these horrible noises,' Gordon said. The vividness with which Gordon experienced the sound in this account is marked by an absence of other available sensory information. Indeed, the sound took on a more affective quality because of the drought in other sensory modalities.

In her discussion of blind aesthetics, Constance Classen describes how, for a blind man standing in a park, the reality of his environment is created out of sound generated by the movements of other people. 'It is precisely when someone else enters the park – when the tread of footsteps is felt, the sound of a voice heard – that the world comes out of nothingness into being' (Classen 1998:141). She draws on the work of the blind writer John Hull, who explains that experience for him is produced through a 'dynamic sequence of sounds', the consequence of a 'world of happenings' (Hull 1990, cited ibid.:142). For Gordon, an alarming and sinister 'world of happenings' on the ward created a haunting reality through sound.

When listening to sounds issuing from behind a privacy curtain, patients are effectively involved in 'acousmatic listening' of a very literal kind (Schaeffer 1966:91). This term is derived from the Greek word *akousmatikoi*, used to refer to the pupils of Pythagoras who were required to listen to their teacher delivering his lectures from behind a veil or screen so that they might better concentrate on his teachings. Schaeffer suggests that in acousmatic listening, auditory attention is focused on sound alone as it becomes disconnected from its (hidden) source. These patients certainly achieve a specific focus on auditory information. Rather than hearing the sounds as disconnected from their source, though, they seem to be involved in an intense imaginative engagement with frightening hidden-yet-vividly-evoked procedures and events.

During my research at the Edinburgh Royal Infirmary I was introduced to a man named Zafer. He explained that he had been admitted to hospital in the UK when, as a seventeen year old, he had been suffering from leukaemia. His condition had quickly worsened and he was soon transferred to a ward where it became clear to him (judging by the condition of the people in neighbouring beds) that he was expected to die. He told me: 'I realized there were two ways out of this ward, the first was to be wheeled out as a corpse, the second was to walk out having made a recovery and essentially beaten the disease.' He prepared himself to 'fight' the disease and save his own life. But the hardest thing to do in preparing his mind and creating a positive outlook, he said, was to shut out the terrible sounds from the patients who were suffering in the beds around him. 'Sounds can kill you,' he told me. They threatened fatally to undermine his concentration on his recovery. He described himself as actually having to preserve what he called a 'space' inside his head where he was determined the sounds should not reach and where his morale could remain unaffected.

In everyday discourse we frequently draw a distinction between an exterior 'physical' and an interior 'mental' space. Above I introduced Cusick's work on the detention camps of the global war on terror. The detainees in her study attempt to escape from excessively loud music played by their torturers and interrogators by retreating into an interior 'mental place'. There is a sense that sounds of all kinds can readily permeate this interiority, influencing mood and affect or, in the case of excessively loud sound, disabling or destabilizing subjectivity altogether. Zafer describes his being forced actively to police and reinforce a boundary between the exterior 'pain-scape' of the ward and the resolved and positive interior space of his own mind (Ellman 1993:101). He considered his success in eventually shutting out the sounds to have been integral to his recovery.

Not all patients to whom I spoke managed to block out the soundscape so well. Some spoke as if the sound within the ward was somehow able to pour itself surreptitiously into the brain through the ear like the poison administered by Claudius in Shakespeare's *Hamlet*. 'It creeps into your headspace,' said a lady who had been in hospital for ten days following a valve replacement operation. Her reference to 'headspace' again indexes a simultaneously physical and mental interior: 'I even hear the ward in my sleep,' she added. Sounds crept into her consciousness at a time when she was incapable of offering resistance. A retired carpenter I interviewed mentioned the Beatles song 'Lady Madonna' which includes the line: 'Lady Madonna, lying on your bed/Listen to the music playing in your head.' 'It's like that in here,' he said. 'The ward plays in your mind.' Again the sound had percolated into the interior space of his thoughts.

During my initial fieldwork period at the Edinburgh Royal Infirmary, *Red Dot Radio* broadcast to patients for three hours each evening. Patients could listen through headphones connected to sockets in the wall. It became clear that *Red Dot Radio* was popular with patients because it provided every day a few hours of relief from the ward soundscape. The ability to escape into a technologically mediated sound world is something generations familiar with personal stereos and MP3 players perhaps take for granted. But the patients I encountered during both research periods tended to be elderly. Few owned personal stereos or were familiar with using them to 'manage' and control their involvement in an external sound environment (Bull 2000).

On most of the beds in the cardiothoracic wards at St Thomas', patients had access to personal media centres. These units, consisting of a screen, control panel, keyboard and telephone receiver, were affixed to the wall beside the beds and could be folded out so that patients could watch television, listen to the radio, search the internet or use the phone from their beds provided they had bought credit. There were headphones that would allow patients to create a degree of privatized auditory space should they desire it. Where available, this unit allowed patients to exercise some control over their own auditory space, or at least, it enabled them to consume a different kind of mediated public soundscape. Patients to whom I spoke appreciated these media centres, but using them was expensive and many older patients found them fiddly and difficult. Also, though patients might immerse themselves in an alternative sound environment quite effectively for a time, ultimately the ward sounds outlasted their attempts at escape.

While, then, distractions were available and could provide some relief, patients would inevitably have to spend time exposed to the sounds around them. They often simply had to do their best to turn a deaf ear. One day as I walked down a ward a patient being attended-to behind a curtain could be heard vomiting profusely. The lady in the adjacent bed was sitting up, turning the pages of a magazine. She held a fixed, bland smile as she pretended to be oblivious to the sounds that were loud and plain. Of course, she had little choice but to do exactly this. Unable to escape the sound, she was obliged to tolerate it as best she could. I felt her facial expression encapsulated the effort made by many simply to put up with the sounds, however invasive, irritating or distasteful. This attempt to remain unperturbed could be understood as itself a way of managing the auditory environment. Like Zafer, patients tried to create privacy through the application of a particular attitude or mental approach, this time one of studied unawareness or indifference (which we could perhaps visualize as mental headphones or earmuffs).

These gestures of 'shutting out' sound or deliberate non-hearing are clearly efforts to resist what Goffman identifies as the 'contaminative exposure' experienced by those entering and living within institutions (1968:31). Introducing this concept, Goffman writes: '[o]n the outside, the individual can hold objects of self-feeling – such as his body, his immediate actions, his thoughts, and some of his possessions, clear of contact with alien and contaminating things. But in total institutions these territories of the self are violated; the boundary that the individual places between his being and the environment is invaded and the embodiments of self profaned' (ibid.:31–2). On the ward, sound can be understood to erode precisely those boundaries between the self and the environment that Goffman considers to be so important to the preservation of a sense of the self. Sound is a powerful agent of contamination, colonizing not only the wider ward space but also the personal space and the interior mental space of many patients.

The notion of contamination is particularly pertinent to the hospital environment where the control of potentially contaminating agents, most obviously pathogens and microbes linked to the spread of disease, is a priority. Indeed, modern medical practices, procedures and buildings are designed with the restriction of this type of contamination in mind. Within the hospital, however, what is taken as contaminative is dependent upon perspective and position. Thus, on certain wards, the presence of medical professionals and visitors represents a contaminative threat to patients, while in other contexts the reverse is true. At times the apparatus needed to combat one form of contamination in hospital only serves to create another. An example of this was provided by the bins that were installed in some of the wards on which I conducted fieldwork. They were pedal operated, meaning that those using them (usually nurses) did not have to risk dirtying their hands. For patients, though, the bins contaminated the ward environment with the noise they made when the pedal was released and the metal lid fell shut with a loud, abrupt bang.

As well as being conscious of the sounds those around them might be making, many of the patients to whom I spoke were acutely aware that they themselves were contributors to the hospital soundscape. They could not only be heard moving around, talking or coughing, but were also obliged to endure more embarrassing forms of auditory exposure. Culturally specific norms of bodily privacy are instilled in people from an early age. In the West it has come to be regarded as inappropriate for other people to see and hear, for instance, certain bodily functions such as hiccupping, burping, farting, being sick or using the toilet. We monitor our own behaviour carefully in this regard, practising self-surveillance, acting in anticipation of listening ears all around us. But hospital patients could do little to guard their acoustic privacy. Intensely 'private' sounds inevitably spilled over into a public space. There was a leakage or seepage of body sounds into spaces occupied by other people (Gunaratnam 2009:7, Lawton 1998). Patients experienced an unpleasant kind of sonic incontinence. Many resented the fact that they could not remove themselves from being in the auditory presence of their neighbours if desired. Not only did they have little control over what sounds intruded into their immediate, personal acoustic space, but also they were limited in their ability to restrict how their own bodies projected into the acoustic space of others.

Conversational space

'It's amazing how many people know about you in here,' said a patient I was chatting to one day. 'Yesterday a doctor I'd never seen before came up to me and started telling me all about myself. In fact he literally knew more about me than I did.' During hospitalization patients are subjected to a range of examinations and investigations that generate information about them. This information, obtained through a variety of techniques and technologies, is circulated through the 'network' of the care system, medical professionals acting on different elements according to their role (Latour 1999, Mol 2002). Knowledge about a patient is both collected in and disseminated through the hospital. Most patients to whom I spoke were perfectly aware of this and knew that information about their bodies that they might once have considered private and sought carefully to control was circulating in a more public discursive zone shared by hospital staff. 'In a way they're all talking about you behind your back,' a lady awaiting a valve transplant told me. 'But there's no point in being precious about it,' she conceded. 'It's got to happen if anything's going to get done.'

There is a sense among doctors, too, that in their comparative vulnerability patients need to be protected from 'raw' medical discourse about their conditions and treatment. They need to be cushioned from the brutality of medical facts and the style of detached clinical objectivity in which those facts are often discussed. The nature of hospital work did mean that while staff might make efforts to keep patients well informed, they also inevitably needed to wait for the results of tests or meetings with other medical professionals before decisions or information could be finalized sufficiently well for that information to be passed on. Patients were not necessarily excluded from decisions regarding their fate, but they also did not necessarily have immediate access to the flows of information through which decisions about diagnosis or treatment were made. Certain kinds of knowledge about patients' bodies needed to remain confidential to doctors, rather than being made known to patients themselves. At the same time, there was often a feeling that information circulating in the zone of clinical discursive space should not be allowed to flow unfiltered back to the patient, or into wider zones occupied by the non-medical public. Most doctors to whom I spoke felt that on the whole, patients should be protected from all but absolutely necessary information about their own cases. They argued that patients would be unlikely to understand medical language, its intricacies and implications. 'A little knowledge is a bad thing,' I was told, and would do patients 'more harm than good.'

Discussions among doctors about patient treatment and care tended to take place away from the wards. They were confined to offices and meeting rooms out of sight and earshot of patients. These might be regarded as the 'corridors of power', the places where medical decisions are made and courses of action planned (Snow 1964). During my fieldwork at St Thomas' Hospital I was able to spend a lot of time in these backspaces. For instance, I attended the Cardiothoracic Unit's weekly meeting where doctors would present cases that had proved particularly interesting or unusual. All those present were doctors and so there was no need to exercise the diplomacy necessary when patients were in the vicinity. There would be occasional jokes about patients, but more striking were remarks that held a straightforward and rather brutal honesty. I am not suggesting that these held any kind of malice. They were merely statements of plain, if sorrowing, fact. For instance, 'This man's going to die fairly soon, isn't he?' In this particular case the patient was a thirty-six-year-old man. It was often strange to meet patients on the wards having overheard conversations of this peculiarly intimate kind about them.

At times, clinically 'private' conversations would spill out of the separate, bounded zone of professional discursive space and into more 'public' spaces within the hospital. This was a danger of which the hospital managers were aware and which they were keen to prevent. In a number of the lifts inside St Thomas' there were signs warning doctors not to talk about patients there lest they be overheard by the patients themselves or concerned friends and relatives who might also be using the lifts. The risks involved in having clinical discussions in inappropriately public spaces were underlined on one occasion when I was with a group of medical students in an empty bed bay. They were working on case notes they were due to present next day, but, distracted from their immediate task, had begun a discussion in which one of the students was criticizing cardiothoracic surgeons. His argument was that these people became highly specialized and expert at one particular procedure or stage of the treatment process. As a consequence, as long as they felt themselves to have done their own work in a satisfactory manner they didn't mind if the patient thereafter lived or died under someone else's care. Of course, what the student said was not fact, and indeed, was not necessarily a view to which he held firmly. I think he was saying this because one of the surgeons had spoken to him harshly in a teaching session the day before and, angered and humiliated, the student wanted to find a way of attacking him in return. However, the group was standing perhaps fifteen metres from a bed where a patient was sitting up talking with a visitor. As the student finished speaking the visitor got up and approached us. 'Excuse me,' she said, 'but my husband has just been told his recent heart bypass operation was unsuccessful. Would you mind having your conversation somewhere else?' After apologizing profusely, the group left.

As the students recognized, their behaviour had been inappropriate. They had not, in this particular case, been discussing a patient but had nonetheless been making unprofessional remarks about the hospital system. To the listening couple the student's words might well have been profoundly upsetting. In all likelihood the student had further undermined the couple's already shaken confidence in those responsible for the surgery. The students belatedly acknowledged the importance of containing their conversations within appropriate conversational zones, not just away from authority figures, but also away from the ward and from patients who might be adversely affected by overhearing what was said.

Of course, doctors would often be required to talk to patients on the wards. At times the subject was not difficult or sensitive and there was no need to speak in confidential tones. But when serious matters had to be discussed the curtain would be drawn around the bed and the doctor(s) would get close to the patient, speaking in a lowered voice, conscious of the need to attempt to generate a zone of private auditory space in a public environment. Their efforts were not always successful. Words and phrases describing particular conditions, giving diagnoses and detailing prognoses were often still audible to other patients. At the time of my fieldwork, the principle that a patient's details should remain confidential to everyone except those immediately involved in his or her care was one of the central tenets of medical practice; sounds (as vocalizations), though, tended to find their way round, under or through this principle, so that private information was once again made public.

The difficulty of creating areas of private conversational space on the wards was well recognized by patients who sometimes found themselves having to hold serious discussions with friends and relatives whilst in hospital. If mobile enough, they would tend to take visitors to the TV room, the landings immediately outside the ward or even the hospital café to get away from those who, albeit unintentionally, might eavesdrop. But patients knew that their neighbours would inevitably overhear a great deal of personal information. A retired army captain I spoke to told me: 'Everyone here is in the strange situation of being a reluctant confidant. They know things about you that you'd rather they didn't and you know things about them that they'd rather you didn't.' An elderly lady I interviewed nodded towards her ward neighbour and said: 'I know what's going on in her heart just as she knows what's going on in mine.' On the ward, just as in the backspace zones of the medical profession, information about their bodies was broadcast, circulated in acoustic and discursive space. This was poignantly illustrated when, as I interviewed a man recovering from bypass surgery, the privacy curtain was pulled around the patient in the bed diagonally opposite his. 'I'm not surprised,' my interviewee said to me in low voice. 'I heard him being told yesterday that the heart muscle's badly damaged. He hasn't got long.'

Sound and unbounded bodies

Within the ward, then, considerable attention was directed towards the control of sonic presences, and the creation and maintenance of zones of private auditory space. I have suggested that efforts in this direction were also often attempts to manage, restrict, or channel the flow of verbally mediated information about patients' bodies: diagnoses, prognoses, treatment details and so on. The communal nature of the ward environment often meant these attempts were only partially successful at best. Bodily interiors were exteriorized through vocalizations that pervaded ward space.

During my research at St Thomas' Hospital I studied the ways in which doctors use and apply auditory knowledge in their day-to-day work. One auditory technique that was frequently adopted during examinations was stethoscopic listening or auscultation. I was struck by the way in which sounds from, for instance, a patient's heart or lungs were brought into the perception of the doctor through the stethoscope. The bodily interior underwent a process of sonic exteriorization. In the case of stethoscopic listening, only the medical professional using the technology is able to hear the sound produced. But modern medical practice also involves the use of other technologies that mediate and externalize internal bodily events through sound.

As indicated in the previous chapter, the repetitive tones produced by electrocardiograph or ECG machines were a noticeable feature of the hospital ward soundscapes I encountered during fieldwork. On the Cardiothoracic Unit at St Thomas', patients were almost invariably suffering from heart problems. Here in particular, electrocardiograph machines were in frequent, if not constant use. Indeed, at the time of my research all patients on these wards received fifteen minutes of electrocardiography twice a day and some were monitored for much longer periods. Patients were conscious of the way that the tones of these machines were part of a much wider medical project to obtain information about the bodily interior. 'They're just part of what they [the doctors] do in here,' one man said, 'which is basically turn you inside out.'

The tones served to transmit information about patients' bodies to the medical professionals on the ward, in particular the nurses. 'It's weird to think that she can hear my heart from all the way over there,' commented one man, gesturing in the direction of a nurse a few beds away, 'but as long as its telling her I'm all right then that's OK.' 'I sometimes get a bit freaked out when this thing is beeping and a nurse walks over,' another patient told me. 'You wonder what it's telling her, what's attracted her attention.' There was an acute awareness too on the part of patients that the tones were irritating and could constitute an intrusion into the auditory space of others. One lady I interviewed was initially reluctant to speak to me and when she eventually agreed told me that she was a shy person. This made being in hospital difficult. She often had to get the nurse's attention in order to ask for things. 'I don't like drawing attention to myself or imposing on people,' she explained. She was reluctant to press the call button to summon assistance and said that receiving attention from numerous members of staff each day made her feel self-conscious. 'As for this thing,' she said, indicating the ECG equipment to which she was attached. 'It's like your heart's shouting.' 'I certainly feel a little bit like I'm on show when it's my heart's beeping away,' another patient remarked. 'But there's nothing you can really do about it. It's just something else we all have to put up with.'

Another technology often used on the wards of the Cardiothoracic Unit was the echocardiograph. In echocardiography or cardiac ultrasound, ultra high frequency sound waves are directed at the heart using a kind of probe known as a 'transducer.' These ultrasound waves (which are of too high a frequency to be audible) are reflected back to the transducer and converted so as to create visual images of the heart on a computer monitor. Echocardiography is a powerful technology and can generate detailed real-time images of the heart as it beats, producing valuable diagnostic information.

Echocardiography often involves the use of Doppler ultrasound. Here, a phenomenon known as the Doppler Effect is exploited in order to make assessments as to whether blood is moving towards or away from the transducer and to gauge the relative velocity of that movement. Some of the reflected sound waves produced using this technique fall within the audible range so that sounds, as well as visual information, are created. A trained technician is able to use these sounds to hear whether, for instance, the blood flow through a certain valve is smooth or turbulent. He or she can also infer the direction of any turbulence present and assess the volume of blood involved. This auditory information is used to guide and direct closer visual inspection. Doppler ultrasound is not crucial to carrying out an echocardiogram, but most sonographers prefer to use the sounds to consolidate their interpretation of the images.

Like the beeps made during electrocardiography, the sounds produced using Doppler ultrasound could be loud, projecting into perceptual space. Intended for the technician, they were also audible to the patient. In several of the ultrasound sessions I observed, patients were captivated by the character of the sound produced by what they usually referred to as 'the echo'. One patient likened it to the rhythmic swishing of a washing machine. Another suggested that it was 'like a ship sinking' with water 'gushing and pouring'. Still another likened the sound to 'water spilling through caves', capturing its swooshing, liquid quality. Mol describes the noise as a '[p]shew pshew, pshew' (2002:60).

Echocardiography was not used as frequently as electrocardiography on the wards in which I conducted research. When necessary, patients were usually transported to a special suite of rooms where a number of echocardiograph machines were located. But when conducted on the wards using a mobile unit, the sounds of echocardiography spilled into the perception of others nearby. 'You're lying there and you can hear the sounds and you're listening and he (the technician) is listening and you know that people on the other side of the curtain, well, they may not be listening but they can hear it too', one patient explained. 'It's an unusual noise so it's bound to attract some attention from those round about', his ward neighbour added. The technicians I spoke to told me that they tended to advise patients that the sounds were unimportant and that no notice should be taken of them. But patients could not help listening and inferring the meaning of the sounds. They tended to interpret them as a direct amplification of events taking place inside their own bodies rather than as sounds generated by a more sophisticated technological process involving the transduction of sound waves reflected off the heart, its tissues and circulating blood. One young man described it as 'like having a microphone in your heart.' Another patient said he found it oddly fascinating hearing his heart 'over the speakers.'

As discussed further in Chapter 7, some patients found listening to the sounds produced during their own echocardiograph scans disturbing. The noises could provoke unsettling imaginative engagements with what they perceived to be internal physiological events. But there seemed to be a general acceptance that the sounds were a necessary part of a diagnostic procedure and that little could be done to prevent them leaking into auditory space. 'I prefer not to have ears cocked in my direction,' said one lady who had undergone many echocardiograms. 'But I don't interfere.' She then employed a phrase I heard used by many patients in relation to a wide variety of medical procedures during my fieldwork: 'In the end you've just got to let them get on with it.'

Mol (2002) emphasizes the importance of keeping actual medical practices, rather than abstract concepts, at the centre of efforts to understand disease. Writing on atherosclerosis, she suggests that the different experts involved in the diagnosis and treatment of this problem (the pathologist, the sonographer, the surgeon, the physiotherapist and so on) all approach different aspects of the disease, and of the patient body, in different ways. For Mol, they enact their own distinct 'versions' or 'variants' of the disease. These clinical 'versions' differ from each other, and differ again in nature and quality from the versions of the disease that are enacted by patients through their own lived experience of the illness and their descriptions of that experience. Mol argues, however, that despite their obvious differences, these distinct versions of the disease (and of the patient body) are able to co-exist simultaneously. In a hospital, she argues, there is not just a single patient body, but rather many versions of the same body: the body is multiple and disease is composite, an entity produced through different versions of the disease and of the body, more or less comfortably 'hanging together' (ibid.:84).

What becomes clear from the accounts given above is that sounds, too, are involved in the production of particular 'versions' of heart disease. There are the sounds of the electrocardiogram that allow the acoustic production of information that is heard by the nurses. There are the sounds of the echocardiogram used by the sonographer to guide his examination of the heart. But these sounds are also heard by the (generally less medically educated and clinically skilled) ears of patients. They constitute part of patients' experience of being ill, so that sounds and listening become involved in what Mol describes as 'lay ways,' as well as professional ways, of 'doing' disease (ibid.:27, 20). We might position electrocardiography and echocardiography as clinical practices through which heart disease is both sounded and enacted at St Thomas' Hospital.

Above I suggested that one dimension of the erosion of privacy which patients experience during hospital stays can be linked to unwanted exposure to sounds from other patients. Privacy can also be threatened when patients lose control over the ways in which their own sounds project into the auditory space occupied by others. But the technologies described above present additional challenges to the patients' auditory control over their own bodies. Electrocardiography and echocardiography have the effect of exteriorizing internal bodily events, amplifying and projecting them into auditory space in unfamiliar acoustic forms. The technologies allow sonically coded information to circulate through the communal diagnostic and discursive space that the ward represents.

Corbin (1994) details changing attitudes towards smells in European thought. He describes how in France in the first half of the eighteenth century, odour became the focus of anxiety around ideas of health and bodily constitution. Smells were (as arguably they still are now) considered to be strongly indicative of corporeal and moral health or decay. In view of the fact that foul smells could emanate from the body, diffusing into the air, it was perceived that 'the body's cement was volatile in nature' (ibid.:17). The body was not conceptualized as solid and self-contained, but as prone to dissipation and flux. The sounds described above also situate the body as potentially diffuse, its internal events seeping and leaking into the perception of others. The body becomes acoustically distributed, an 'unbounded' or 'boundless' entity (Lawton 1998, Rice 2008a).

Haraway introduces the notion of the cyborg, which she describes as 'a hybrid of machine and organism' (1991:149). Medical professionals might be regarded as cyborgs in the way that they form couplings with machines in order to go about their work of diagnosing, monitoring and managing illness. At the same time, patients on hospital wards may be positioned as cyborgs through their being connected to machines at various stages during their care. Indeed, Haraway indicates that modern medicine is 'full of cyborgs' (ibid.:150, 171–2). She goes on to ask: 'Why should our bodies end at the skin, or include at best other things encapsulated by skin?' (ibid.:178). The concept of the cyborg allows bodies to be extended through fusion with machines so that the boundaries marking each as distinct from the other become unclear or dissolve altogether. An important characteristic of the sonic cyborgs produced by the unions of people and medical technology described above is their capacity to produce and attend to sounds. They indicate that bodies may be extended beyond the skin not simply through their fusion with machines, but through the sounds generated in the process of that fusion.

The body broadcast

In the comparatively public spaces of wards of the public hospitals in which my fieldwork took place, sounds created persistent threats to the preservation of patients' privacy. Cusick (2013) suggests that the detainees in her study attempted to find refuge from the loud sounds to which they were subjected by retreating inside themselves. They might put their fingers in their ears, trying to seal off and preserve some vestige of physical and mental space. In the surveillance-intense setting of the detention centre the only privacy available to detainees seems to have been inside this mental space, which was invaded and at times even annihilated by the intensity of the loud music. In a similar way, some patients emphasized the difficulty of preserving an interior 'headspace' in an institutional environment in which they were in uncomfortable sonic proximity to others. But stays in hospital were fraught with anxieties over not only intrusive sounds, but also the sounds they themselves were likely to make. Patients had an acute awareness of the need for self-surveillance, concealment and quietening. As the discussion of electrocardiography and echocardiography suggests, the sounds of diagnostic and monitoring technologies could also create or exacerbate a perceived inability to control and police bodily boundaries. Sounds sometimes constituted 'a problem to the borders of the self', moving across them in unsettling ways (Bubandt 1998:65).

In the context described above, the notion of privacy seems to imply a capacity to manage the extent and nature of auditory intrusions into a zone of intimate or close 'personal space'. It also refers to an ability to determine the extent of one's own acoustic presences within a space. We can imagine roughly concentric zones of auditory space radiating away from the body, each carrying a relative (and culturally particular) charge reflecting a degree of personal ownership, occupancy and agency. But living within the institutional setting of a hospital (and in particular the cardiothoracic unit) and being subjected to the routines and practices in place there, many of the patients to whom I spoke clearly felt that the integrity of the body as a core private space was, at times, challenged. The body could no longer be understood as being located at the spatial centre of a set of concentric rings. Indeed, through sounds, bodily interiors were exteriorized in many ways on the wards, and these exteriorizations were re-internalized through different sets of listening ears so that it became difficult to be certain any more where bodily boundaries (and thus related zones of 'owned' 'occupied' or 'controlled' space) began and ended. As it is sonically broadcast, the body becomes dispersed, dissipated. Indeed, sounds – words, whispers, coughs, cries, beeps, whooshes

– encourage us to reflect on the multiplicity of sonic forms in which the body and information about the body can travel. In an institution such as a large public hospital, sound makes the materiality of the body both multiple and transmissible across spatial, social and moral boundaries; 'flows' of these sounds draw our attention to the constant shifting and morphing of bodily space. They emphasize in turn the fragility and fluidity of public and private space as constructed and experienced by patients.

This chapter draws upon material from Tom Rice 'Broadcasting the body: the 'private' made 'public' in hospital soundscapes', in Georgina Born (ed.) *Music, Sound and Space: Transformations of Public and Private Experience.* Cambridge University Press (2013). Reproduced with permission.

CHAPTER 3

Acoustemology of the Body

A Brief History of Diagnostic Listening

The two previous chapters have been concerned with patient experiences of hospital soundscapes. Both have indicated, however, that sound and listening, as well as being integral to patient experiences of the hospital, can also be important in the generation and mediation of medical knowledge. In the chapters that follow, the focus shifts to applications of listening and particularly stethoscopic listening in medical practice. This chapter examines the roots of Western medicine's appropriation of sounds in the mediation of internal bodily processes and states. It explores how, historically, medical practitioners have listened to the body and have worked to render it acoustically intelligible.

In *The Birth of the Clinic*, Foucault (1973) identifies the turn of the eighteenth century as a point of transition in the way in which doctors attempted to understand illness (ibid.:xii). The focus of medical knowledge practices was shifting, which also entailed changes in the relationship between the doctor and the patient. Doctors were moving away from a preoccupation with the interpretation of symptoms as related by patients. They were instead becoming increasingly concerned with anatomy and pathology. This change was accompanied by an enthusiasm for dissection (Reiser 1997:828). Richardson (1987) writes that in the early nineteenth century there was a huge demand for corpses to be made available for this purpose. Medical interest was redirected from the patient, the bearer of a subjectively organized disease, to the body, a site of layers and surfaces that could be rendered visible to the doctor through dissection. For Foucault, this notion of visibility is crucial. Vision, and the exercise of the gaze, was integral to the anatomical drive in medicine.

Foucault does recognize that the non-visual senses, and particularly techniques of listening and touching were also used to engage with the body during the anatomical turn. For him, 'the medical gaze embraces more than is said by the word "gaze' alone" (1973:165). It comprises, Foucault suggests, a 'sensory triangulation' or 'sight/touch/hearing trinity' (ibid.:164, 165). The medical gaze possesses a 'pluri-sensorial structure' (ibid.). It is a gaze that touches and hears, as well as sees. But though he gives more than a passing nod to the importance of listening and touching, Foucault allows a concern with seeing to dominate his archaeology of modern medical knowledge. An 'absolute, absolutely integrating gaze' provides the meta-sense of medical perception (ibid.:167).

While Foucault's work on the gaze has become a key reference for anthropological work on medicine, this chapter aims to demonstrate that 'listening is a central component of the genealogy of medical modernity' (Sterne 2003b:191). In doing so, it does not situate listening and gazing as irreconcilable or opposing sensory categories. It recognizes that there is considerable literal and metaphorical interplay between hearing and seeing in medical work. For example, while referring to an acoustic technology, the word 'stethoscope' implies visual examination. 'Steth' is derived from the Greek word *stethos* meaning 'chest'. 'Scope' comes from a Latin ending derived from the Greek *skopein*, meaning to look at or examine. This ending has been used to form a number of other words denoting scientific instruments that enable the making of observations, for instance, 'laryngoscope' and 'otoscope'. The word 'stethoscope', then, refers to a device used to see through listening. While recognizing synergies between hearing and seeing, however, this chapter accentuates the role that the former has played historically in the production of medical knowledge.

The chapter gives a brief history of techniques of diagnostic listening, focusing in particular on the origin and development of stethoscopic listening or mediate auscultation, the practice which is the focus of the rest of this book. It explains how and why auscultation came to be integrated into Western medical practice, thereby providing important background for the chapters that follow. But it also makes the point that the development of mediate auscultation involved a reconfiguration of the patient body, allowing it to become acoustically intelligible to a far greater extent than had been possible using previous medical listening techniques. At the same time, because mastering the use of the stethoscope required considerable training and practice, mediate auscultation brought about a reconfiguration of the bodies of medical students and doctors, which were positioned as entities whose auditory capacities must be shaped and trained. Medical men needed to become good listeners. As auscultation entered routine use and doctors were increasingly expected to be familiar with the technique, the bodies of doctors became subject to a further reconfiguration, becoming positioned as the repositories of valuable specialist auditory knowledge and skill. The chapter indicates that auscultation was closely linked to the development of social status and distinction for physicians, pointing to the co-production of a specialist medical aurality and medical professionalization.

In an article entitled 'The body's career in anthropology', Csordas (1999) attempts to detail the different ways in which the discipline has engaged with the body. In his thorough review he notes the presence of work on the senses. He mentions that important studies have highlighted cultural elaborations of smell, taste and sound, and references Classen *et al.* (1994), Stoller (1997) and Feld (1990) respectively. Csordas emphasizes anthropologists' attention to the sensory capabilities of the body, and through Feld refers to its capacity to hear. But Feld's work on the Kaluli also emphasizes that the body itself is a reverberant space. The Kaluli identify a correspondence between the resonant flow of the voice through the body (reverberating, for example, in the abdomen, chest, throat and head) and the resonant flow of water through the landscape (1996:96–101). By exploring practices of medical listening, this chapter also underscores the body's dual acoustic nature, not only as sonically sensitive, but also as sonically productive. It emphasizes both the auditory receptivity and the sonorousness of the body, taking a step towards developing the body's sonic 'career in anthropology'.

Ways to listen

Medical practitioners have evidently used the sounds of the body as clues to the health of its interior for centuries. Mangione indicates that references are made to the diagnostic significance of breath sounds in the Ebers papyrus (c. 1500 BC) and the Hindu Vedas (c. 1400–1200 BC) (2000:295). In the fourth century BC, however, Hippocrates described a practice that came to be known as 'immediate auscultation', which involved pressing an ear to the patient's body in order to listen to the internal sounds (ibid; Marks 1972:19–20). Among the doctors whose teaching sessions I attended, Hippocrates was considered to have pioneered the use of listening as a way of gathering information about specific events in the bodily interior. Hippocrates is also known to have practised a technique known as 'succussion' (Reiser 1978:21). This involved actively agitating the patient's body, shaking it whilst listening for a splash that might indicate the presence of fluid in the chest cavity, a sound now known as the 'Hippocratic succussion splash' (Fleming 1997:87).

Doctors continued to practise immediate auscultation as the centuries progressed, and the technique was still in use in the early nineteenth century. Fleming (ibid.) and Lachmund (1999) argue that the practice was not abandoned until much later. Though I never saw it being applied during my fieldwork, the image below from 1953 of blind doctor Albert-Andre Nast listening to a baby by pressing an ear to its back suggests that immediate auscultation was still used by some doctors in certain contexts and had not completely disappeared from medical practice even in the mid-twentieth century. Succussion seems to have received little use as a medical technique in later years, perhaps because it seems counter-intuitive to shake vigorously anyone feeling fragile because he or she is unwell! However, contemporary medical students still learn that when a hernia allows water to leak into the chest cavity it is possible to hear a 'succussion splash' as the patient's torso moves. Also, the sloshing normally heard when the stomach is moved immediately after a large liquid meal is known as an 'abdominal succussion splash.' It is taken as a sign of gastric retention or obstruction if heard at times other than after meals.

Hippocrates, then, is known to have used sounds as clues to the condition of the bodily interior. However, Reiser suggests that it was Robert Hooke who first grasped the scope and diagnostic potential of auscultation when he wrote:

> There may be . . . a Possibility of discovering the Internal Motions and Actions of Bodies by the sound they make, who knows but that as in a Watch we may hear the beating of the Balance, and the running of the Wheels, and the striking of the Hammers and the grating of the Teeth, and Multitudes of other Noises; who knows, I say, but that it may be possible to discover the Motions of the Internal Parts of Bodies, whether Animal, Vegetable or Mineral, by the sound they make, that one may discover the Works perform'd in the several Offices and Shops of a Man's body, and thereby discover what Instrument or Engine is out of order. (Hooke 1705:39–40, cited Reiser 1978:23).

Sketching what must at the time have been a futuristic micro-acoustics, Hooke conceptualizes the body as productive of a set of sounds that reference specific parts and processes of its physiology and function. As later became apparent, '[d]ifferent things make different sounds. The air going in and out of the lungs makes one sound. Blood pumping through the heart makes still another sound. Liquid passing through the kidneys makes still another sound' (Marks 1972:16).

A further technique for the use of sounds in diagnosis is thought to have emerged in 1761 when Leopold Auenbrugger hit upon the idea of percussion. This is perhaps best described as an 'audile-tactile' method of examination (Sterne 2003a:119). Rather than simply listening to corporeal processes and events, it involves striking the body in order to make the spaces formed or enclosed by tissues and organs resonate. Auenbrugger was an innkeeper's son

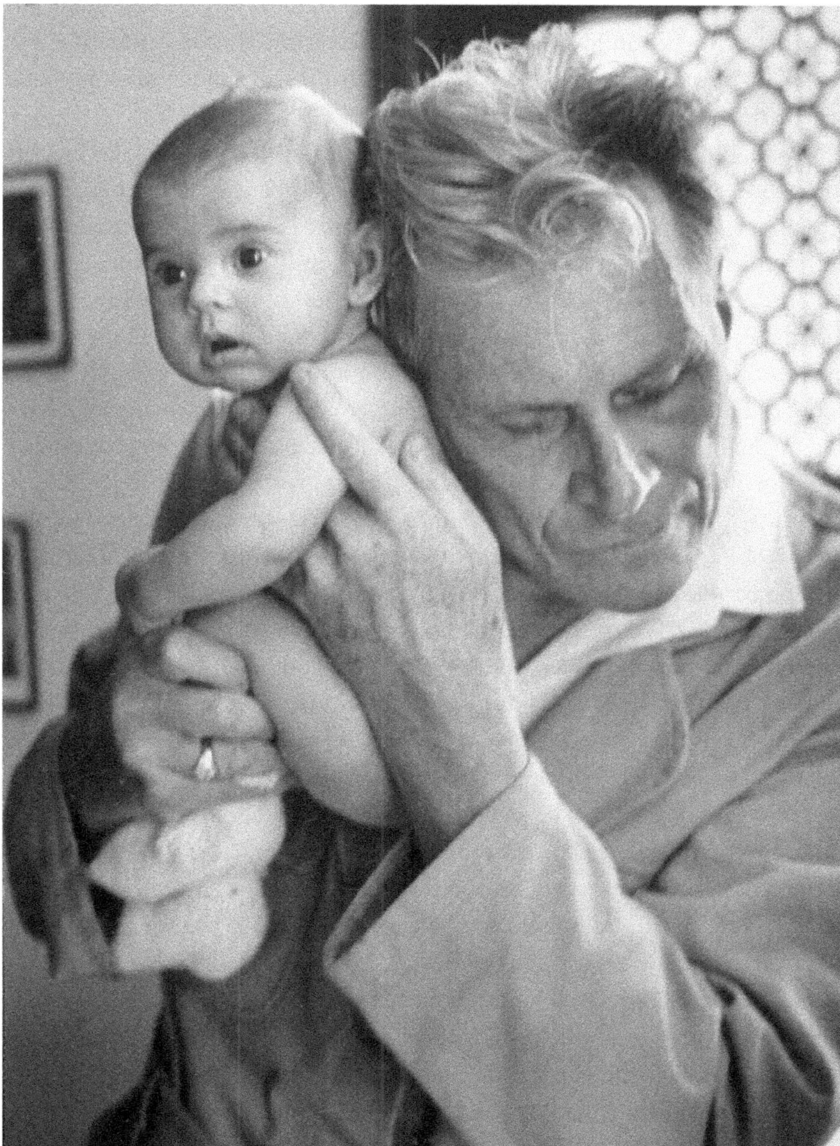

Figure 1 *Blind doctor Albert-Andre Nast using his ear instead of a stethoscope, Chelles, France. 1953. Photograph by Thomas MacAvoy. Time LIFE collection. Used with permission.*

and as a child had learned to test the fullness of barrels by thumping them (Porter 1997:256). Switching kegs for rib cages, he noted that if struck with a finger, healthy and unhealthy chests produced different sounds: 'a healthy chest sounded like a cloth-covered drum . . . a muffled sound or one of high pitch indicated pulmonary disease' (ibid.). Porter writes that Auenbrugger's work attracted little attention when it first appeared. It was not until after the charismatic physician Jean Corvisart published a French translation of it and began to apply and teach percussion himself that the technique gained general acceptance (ibid.:308).

Percussion remains an important technique in the clinical examination. The students with whom I studied were taught that, as Auenbrugger had attempted to demonstrate, percussive sounds are resonant over aerated spaces and dull in those where there is fluid. As part of the chest examination, for instance, students were taught to percuss the lungs. They would tap (using the middle finger of one hand to knock on the second phalange of the middle finger of the other) at an upper, middle, and lower point on each side of the patient's back and on top of the shoulder. Percussion was also applied to the abdomen to determine whether abdominal distension, if present, involved solids or liquids (producing dull sounds) or gas (producing resonant ones). As well as practising on patients' bodies, students would often try to perfect the knack of getting a really good resonance by tapping on walls and other surfaces, as well as their own bodies. Sinclair describes the way in which the students he studied at University College Hospital would practise finding where the supports of tables were by 'percussing out' their tops (1997:209).

One case in fieldwork demonstrated clearly the way in which percussion can show up a particular problem. During a morning of consultations, an elderly man entered the room accompanied by a woman who introduced herself as his daughter. The daughter explained that she was very worried about her father. He lived in a home for the elderly and she was only able to see him monthly. Over recent visits, however, she thought she had seen a rapid decline in his health. Although he said he did not feel too bad, she believed he was only saying this so as not to worry her. The man himself did not offer any comment. Dr Coltart asked him to remove his top things and lie on the couch and said he would examine him. It was easy to see as he undressed that he was very thin and this visibly upset his daughter. Dr Coltart conducted a thorough examination. When he had finished he asked the man if he would mind if we took turns to percuss his back as he sat forward. The man said he didn't and added jokingly that he 'liked an audience'. Clearly worried that asking us to percuss meant Dr Coltart had found something serious, the daughter's eyes filled with tears, and I noticed that she looked closely at each of our faces as we percussed, searching for any signs that might give away the seriousness of what we heard. When my turn came I pressed the middle finger of my left hand flat against the man's back, knocking on it with the middle finger of my right hand. I percussed at six points: three on each side, at the upper, middle and lower areas. On the left side, a resonant sound was produced, suggesting that the lung was clear and healthy. On the right side the upper percussions were also resonant. The lower percussions on the right side, however, were definitely dull. The contrast with the left side and the upper right was striking, and suggested there was fluid in the right lower lung. When the man was dressed, Dr Coltart explained to him and his daughter what he had found. The daughter began to cry when Dr Coltart explained that he thought it would be best to admit her father to hospital straight away to remove the fluid and find out what was causing it to accumulate. After they left the consultation room carrying the forms Dr Coltart had given them, he told us that he was sure the man had cancer.

An invention story

During an early teaching session I attended, Dr Coltart asked his students 'Who invented the stethoscope?' None of us knew. He then gave the inventor's name as Rene Theophile Hyacinth Laennec. Laennec evidently knew of and admired Auenbrugger's work on percussion. The practice was, he felt, 'one of the most valuable discoveries with which medicine has ever been enriched' (Laennec 1846:2). Laennec shared Auenbrugger's empiricist orientation to diagnosis, but he felt that percussion was limited in its scope, accuracy and reliability. He observed that it gave an indication only of fullness and emptiness, and wrote that: 'we frequently stand in need of a more constant and certain sign than that furnished by percussion' (ibid.:2–3). Laennec was also familiar with immediate auscultation (it was practised by his colleague Gaspard Bayle), and it surprised him that the technique described by Hippocrates had never been more fully and systematically explored (Reiser 1997:828). Nonetheless, he considered the practice to be unsatisfactory in many ways. Because it involved direct contact between the ear and the patient's chest, it had some value as a tactile means of discerning the pulsations of the heart, but Laennec felt it to be 'alike inconvenient to the physician and the patient; its disagreeableness alone often renders it almost impracticable in hospitals' (ibid.). It is easy to understand the repugnance that might be provoked by pressing one's ear to the chest of a patient 'who may be dirty or bathed in perspiration' (ibid.:21). Laennec also wrote of immediate auscultation that: 'it can hardly be proposed to females in general, and in some the large size of the mammae presents an insuperable obstacle to its adoption' (ibid.:3). Not only was immediate auscultation often impracticable on women; for a Frenchman in the early nineteenth century it required an unacceptable level of intimacy with them.

Dr Coltart told his students how one day in 1816, Laennec was walking through the Tuileries Garden in Paris. The case of one of his patients, a young woman suffering from a heart condition, was playing on his mind. He had been unable to learn anything about her problem from the accounts she gave. The fact that she was female and considerably overweight also made immediate auscultation impracticable. While he was wondering what to do, Laennec saw a group of children playing around a log that was sitting on top of a pile of rubbish. The children at one end of the log were pressing their ears to the wood. They seemed to be able to hear the knocks and scratches made by the children at the other end. This was Laennec's 'Eureka!' moment. He returned immediately to his patient at the Necker Hospital. Rolling a book into a tight cylinder so that it resembled a log, he pressed it to her heart and found he could hear her heartbeat clearly.

I heard Dr Coltart repeat this story to other groups of students, and, indeed, it can be found in several texts (e.g. Marks 1972, Welsby, Parry and Smith 2003). It was being passed on, reproduced in new generations of doctors as an accepted if generally unscrutinized creation myth for a now ubiquitous piece of medical technology. Others writing on the invention of the stethoscope are less specific as to what took place. Reiser states that Laennec simply 'recalled the well-known acoustic phenomenon: that sound was augmented when it travelled through solid bodies, as when a scratch noise made at one end of a piece of wood can be heard at the other end' (1997:828). He does not specify what caused Laennec to make this recollection. Fleming goes as far as to declare that '[t]here is... no documentary support for the attractive traditional story that it was the sight of children at play, scratching one end of a log of wood and listening at the other in the courtyard of the Louvre, which first gave Laennec the idea of mediate auscultation' (1997:88). However, while he aims to discredit the myth, Fleming in fact only reproduces the 'attractive traditional story' by referring to it in such detail.

It is unclear exactly where Laennec's inspiration for the stethoscope came from. But though Sterne argues that he may well have crafted the story with the benefit of hindsight, Laennec himself relates how, sitting at the bedside of a young female patient whose gender and obesity made immediate auscultation useless, he rolled a stack of paper into a cylinder and pressed it to his patient's heart (Sterne 2003a:102, Laennec 1846:4). He was pleased to find how well his first impromptu stethoscope worked: 'I...was alike surprised and gratified to hear the pulsations of the heart much more clearly and distinctly than I had ever heard them by the immediate application of the ear' (ibid.). The process of listening with what Laennec later called the 'stethoscope', 'pectriloque' or 'cylinder' (Sterne suggests it also had many other names) became known as *l'auscultation mediate* (2003a:104). This served to differentiate the new technique from immediate auscultation as a form of listening mediated by an instrument (Lachmund 1999:424).

A number of historians of medicine have observed that mediate auscultation developed during a time of profound change in the medical profession, namely the anatomical turn identified above (Porter 1997, Reiser

1997, Fleming 1997). Laennec's belief that mediate auscultation offered indications like those furnished to a surgeon suggests that he considered the route to true medical knowledge to be through opening up the body, allowing its mysteries be revealed to the perception of the doctor (1846:4). Laennec's key method in developing the technique of mediate auscultation was entirely in keeping with the enthusiasm for anatomy in the wider medical culture of his day. He would listen to the chests of patients admitted to his hospital, carefully noting what he heard. He would continue to listen as the disease progressed and then, when the patient died, would conduct a dissection and observe the physiological effects the disease had brought about. For example, in his 'Case 29: Metallic tinkling in a vast Tuberculous Excavation half converted into Fistula,' Laennec explains that a fifty-year-old washerwoman, Marianne Levas, was admitted to the Necker Hospital having experienced an acute worsening of the cough from which she had suffered for many years (ibid.:319). He writes that:

> On applying the stethoscope to the antero-superior part of the right side of the chest, as well as under the right armpit, a distinct pectoriloquy was heard. There was likewise observed when the patient coughed or spoke, and especially when she respired, a tinkling similar to that of a small bell just ceasing to ring, or of a fly buzzing in a china vase (ibid.:320).

Laennec diagnosed a 'vast tuberculous excavation occupying the whole superior lobe of the right lung, and containing a small quantity of fluid tubercles, especially in the summit of the left lung, and at the root of the right' (ibid.). He was obliged to send the patient home four days after her admission on account of her disruptive behaviour, but she was re-admitted a month later and Laennec writes that he detected exactly the same signs with the stethoscope. She died after a further two weeks, and Laennec conducted a post-mortem twenty-four hours after her death. Laennec's diagnosis was confirmed when, on cutting open the right lung, he noted: 'the superior half of this lung was occupied by an extremely large excavation, containing about two spoonfuls only of a liquid, yellow, puriform matter' (ibid.:321). This cavity was sufficiently large to 'have received the fist of the stoutest man' (ibid.). Through repeated observations of this nature, Laennec was able to generate a large body of work detailing the audible signs of tuberculosis and other diseases, and showing how these signs reflected physiological changes inside the body. It is worth noting the synergy of listening and visual observation here. Sounds are situated as signs of underlying physiology and pathology, but their origin and import is established by visual observations made during dissection.

Following his systematic listening and referencing of sounds to organic changes, Laennec was able to identify sounds that were characteristic of particular pathologies. Thus, for instance, upon auscultating a woman who had been complaining of a cough, Laennec describes how he was surprised to be able to detect a specific area in which her voice seemed to sound directly in his ear (ibid.:31). He found this particular acoustic phenomenon, which he called 'pectoriloquism' (and which he also detected in the case of Marianne Levas described above), in around twenty other patients, most of whom were known to be or suspected of being in the advanced stages of tuberculosis but some of whom initially seemed healthy. Laennec later autopsied these patients and found lesions characteristic of tuberculosis in all of them. He was thus able to deduce that, even in those who were apparently healthy, a pectoriloquism was a reliable sign that tuberculosis was present (ibid.).

The technique of mediate auscultation ultimately meant the physician could interrogate the body of the patient while he or she was still alive. The stethoscope allowed Laennec to access a set of signs that informed him of the condition of the organs within and it was no longer necessary for patients to die (though clearly they very frequently did) in order for anatomization to take place. Auscultation created scope for the 'autopsy of the living', and could be used to make informed predictions about the presence, absence, or the progress of disease in the living patient (Sterne 2003b). Indeed, the technique was predicated on the body being animate, for only then would it produce the sounds necessary for diagnosis.

An acoustemology of the body

Prior to the anatomical turn, medical practice had been based on the doctor listening to a patient relate his or her symptoms, forming a diagnosis from what he had understood. But like Auenbrugger, Laennec wanted to be able to make diagnoses by recourse to his own senses. The two men shared the belief that disease should be assessed through the rational consideration of empirically valid signs. For Laennec, the sounds of the body were precisely these, voices that did not lie and could not deceive. The doctor could listen to them and form an independent opinion of their significance. Auscultation situated the body as eloquent irrespective of its owner's capacity to speak. Through its sounds, the body was richly and truthfully descriptive of itself and of its interior spaces. Medical aurality, then, was redirected and reconfigured. The doctor was less an interpreter of words and increasingly an interrogator of the body, forming clinical judgements based on his independent assessment of diagnostic signs. Sterne suggests that in the nineteenth century the stethoscope became emblematic of this modern clinical approach (2003a:136).

It was indicated above that the stethoscope was partly 'born out a desire... to separate the physician from the patient' (Salomon 2001:56). Foucault describes the stethoscope as 'solidified distance' (1973:164). The instrument 'authorizes a withdrawal' (ibid.). It is the materialization of a step back, made partly in revulsion and partly in the interests of propriety and decorum. But for Sterne, the significance of the distance between the doctor and patient that the stethoscope allows is perceptual as much as spatial. The instrument makes 'distance between knower and known' (2003b:196). It reflects the doctor's disengagement from all but the signs given by the body of the patient, which in auscultation manifest themselves as sounds. The listener can obtain an objective, detached, carefully focused form of auditory concentration. The stethoscope creates a distinct perceptual space, amplifying the sounds of the body, allowing the doctor to operate in the 'sonorous clarity of reason and rationality' (2003a:136).

It is clear that auscultation, as much as allowing physicians to hear sounds from inside the patient body, also produced a particular 'body' of sounds. The practice permitted sounds to be heard in such a way that they could be encountered as discrete acoustic objects. Individual noises could be isolated, separated and objectified as diagnostic signs. They could be closely referenced to specific areas of the organs in which they had their origin and be systematically schematized as indicators of pathological states or changes in the body. Laennec described, often in extraordinary detail, a variety of pathological sounds: the pectriloquism, the moist crepitous rattle, the mucous or gurgling rattle, the dry sonorous rattle, the dry sibilous rattle, the dry crepitous rattle, utricular buzzing and amphoric resonance to name just a few (ibid.:125).

Perceived through the stethoscope, the soundscape of the body is characterized by flow and by recurrent patterns of movement: of blood around the body and through the vessels and chambers of the heart, of breath in and out of the lungs, of matter and gases through the gut. Of course auscultation also allows the detection of sounds produced by contact or friction in the body. A pleural rub, for example, which can occur in patients with pneumonia, is created when thickened, roughened surfaces rub together as the lungs expand and contract. The sounds that constitute the heartbeat are made by the snapping closure of the heart valves. Broadly speaking, however, as Sterne suggests, auscultation creates a 'hydraulic hermeneutics, charting the motions of liquids and gases through the body' (2003b:203). Flows of air or fluid, shaped by the widening or narrowing of openings, the hardening or softening of tissue, describe the spaces of the living body.

Feld (1996) details how the Kaluli have a specialized knowledge of the sounds of the visually inaccessible rainforest environment in which they live. He identifies their system of engagement with these sounds as an 'acoustemology', whereby 'sound is central to making sense, to knowing, to experiential truth' (1996:97). He describes the Kaluli's intimate knowledge of the sounds made by the rivers and creeks that flow steeply downwards through their territory, and considers sonic sensitivity to be central to Kaluli 'sense and sensuality of emplacement' (ibid.). Laennec was also producing a specialized sonic knowledge, an acoustemology of patterns of flow through the visually obscured space of the bodily interior. Rather than an 'acoustemology of place', though, he produced an acoustemology of the body. Given that it was the stethoscope that allowed him to hear body sounds that had never been heard before, we might consider Laennec to have created what Greene and Porcello (2005) describe as a 'technostemology' or technologically mediated acoustemology of the body.

Later doctors would continue to confirm, challenge and reappraise Laennec's research and his lexicon of sounds as diagnostic signs. For instance, following extensive engagement with Laennec's ideas and findings, Joseph Skoda, key proponent of what Lachmund terms the 'Viennese approach', who worked a great deal on auscultation in the 1830s and 40s, argued that rather than being directly referenced to specific underlying pathologies, sounds should instead first be described by reference to the acoustic principles that determined their particular character. At the same time Skoda sought to reorganize and simplify Laennec's lexicon of auscultatory signs, which often depended upon the making of very subtle auditory distinctions and differentiations (Lachmund 1999). It also later became clear that Laennec had misunderstood the specifics of the cardiac cycle, and had therefore made errors concerning the import of some heart sounds. As medical knowledge and understanding of the anatomy and function of the human body developed, however, sounds could be indexed to specific physiological events or changes and linked to particular diseases with greater certainty. Over time doctors' acoustic understanding of the body became wider, deeper and more precise. Ongoing research and a steadily improving understanding of human anatomy and physiology, as well as modifications in stethoscope design, meant that auscultation as a technique became increasingly reliable and expedient.

As well as being a pioneer of mediate auscultation, Laennec was an originator and innovator in terms of the technology the practice required. According to Marks, soon after his initial improvisation with a tube of paper Laennec 'bought a woodworking lathe, taught himself how to operate it, and began to make cylinders…with various diameters and lengths' (1972:29). He settled on a monaural (one-eared) device, essentially a simple wooden cylinder, but later made improvements and alterations, adding, for instance, a funnel shape at one end which he found allowed lung sounds to be heard better. This funnel could be stopped with a plug with a small hole through the centre which was of the same diameter as that in the rest of the tube, and which Laennec found better for listening to voice or heart sounds (ibid.:31–2). Other variations included alterations to allow the stethoscope to be unscrewed into two parts to enhance its portability. Laennec also experimented with materials such as glass, metal and even a thin material of beaten gold known as 'gold-beater's skin', but found these to be less satisfactory than light wood, the material in which stethoscopes continued to be made for more than a century (1846:5).

Laennec's early stethoscope underwent many developments as later doctors built on its principle. The 'candlestick design', with a funnel base, slender stem and a flared top for the doctor's ear, proved popular and was manufactured into the 1870s (Marks 1972:36). To counter the inflexible wooden design, various instruments were later produced which were made of pliant tubing (Reiser 1978:40–1). Although conceptualized before this date, the first successful binaural model appeared in 1851. This design promised greater acoustic sensitivity and clarity (ibid.:41). In 1855, Dr George Philip Camman of New York City published a design that used flexible rubber tubing to conduct the sound from a single chest piece into two earpieces. This stethoscope was light and could be carried easily, and the rubber tubes meant the instrument could be folded into a pocket. It became a standard design and was mass-produced (ibid.). By 1855, then, the stethoscope was in more or less its modern form. One important change, however, has been made since that time. The chest piece, which was formerly of a 'bell' design like the funnel of Laennec's monaural stethoscope, had proved good for detecting the lower, rumbling body sounds, but did not pick up higher-pitched sounds effectively. Consequently, a diaphragm, a disc of taut material that responds to high frequency sound vibrations, was added. On most modern stethoscopes, the diaphragm forms one side of the chest piece and the bell the other. It is easy to alternate quickly between the two. This type of stethoscope has come to be carried and used so routinely by doctors that it is now widely recognized as the symbol of the medical profession.

Doctors as listeners

As well as producing a new instrument for accessing the sounds of the body, and a new body of sounds as diagnostic signs, Laennec's technique enabled and indeed demanded a particular kind of listening. Auscultation required auditory attention to be carefully channelled and focused. It necessitated some theoretical and factual knowledge of how sounds could correspond to physiological changes in the body interior, but it also required that the doctor apply himself to attaining practical knowledge of what was and still is generally regarded as a demanding skill. Anyone who wanted to be a competent auscultator would have to learn to handle and place the stethoscope correctly and to identify a range of sounds requiring often very fine acoustic differentiations. This ability could not be learned from books but required a practical apprenticeship.

Laennec produced a treatise on the diagnosis of diseases of the chest which he first published in 1819, issuing a revised version in 1826. Keen to learn the technique for themselves, doctors would travel to France in order to receive instruction from Laennec (Fleming 1997:90). In describing the adoption of stethoscopic listening by medical practitioners it is important to avoid reproducing what Latour describes as 'diffusionist' narratives, whereby technologies spread as if by their own volition through the static medium of society (1987:136). Auscultation did not flow between medical communities through the funnel of a text tradition, nor was it merely a question of technology transfer by which the stethoscope was simply taken to other countries. Rather, auscultation as a skill was carried between communities of medical practitioners.

Writing specifically on the use of the stethoscope, Maulitz argues that the importation of the French anatomico-pathological tradition into England was a process in which '*experience*, from the dissection table and the hospital wards, flowed through the careers of multitudinous young Englishmen as they made the journey out and back...The year in France was, far from a passive period of observation, a veritable *tour de main*' (1987:136 original italics). It was also a *tour d'oreille*, a time in which young doctors could practise and perfect the new skills the technique of auscultation demanded using an 'ears on' approach (Lachmund 1999:440). Laennec was evidently an energetic teacher, instructing numerous students and young doctors. Fleming writes that 'Laennec kept records of his foreign visitors, sometimes with comments on their talent for auscultation. The performance of, for instance, Thomas Hodgkin, who introduced the stethoscope to Guy's Hospital, was recorded as no better than '*assez bien*,' (1997:90). A certain Charles Williams was more impressive; he is recorded as having been '*tres bien*' (ibid.). Auscultation, then, did not only configure the patient body as a dynamic acoustic space amenable to interpretation: it could also be understood to involve a reconfiguration of the perceptual skills of medical students and young doctors, requiring that they take on new auditory sensitivities and capabilities. As Sterne observes, '[a] skilled doctor had to have a highly developed sense of hearing' (2003b:214).

Furst writes that 'it would be erroneous to jump to the conclusion that the stethoscope was rapidly hailed and assimilated into general practice' (1998:57). Instead, the 'adoption of the stethoscope was patchy' (ibid.). Lachmund (1999) and Nicolson (2004) indicate that Laennec's ideas were variously accepted, contested and subjected to re-evaluation by communities of doctors in major centres of medical practice across Europe. Lachmund explores two distinct (though clearly related) approaches to auscultation and the interpretation of body sounds that emerged in Paris and Vienna during the nineteenth century. But although approaches to, skill in, and enthusiasm for auscultation would continue to vary between medical communities and their individual members, the technique was normalized and ultimately became routine in medical practice. Sterne writes that 'stethoscopy was everywhere' by the end of the nineteenth century (2003b:192). He indicates that practitioners who did not use auscultation at that time risked their professional reputations (ibid.). The ability to practise auscultation was synonymous with modern medical professionalism.

Those patients who were among the first to encounter the stethoscope were evidently disconcerted by the level of intrusion that its use required, and many feared the instrument, assuming it would cause pain (Reiser 1997:831–2). Equally, they were disturbed by the physical intimacy that the technique demanded. Because the examination was a new development, patients were unused to it and found the process awkward (ibid.:832). But they were also amazed by the stethoscope's powers, and the reliable manner in which it appeared to describe their conditions to the doctor (ibid.). In Wells's famous story *The Country of the Blind*, the main character, Nunez, stumbles upon a village inhabited entirely by blind people. He is awed to find that the members of this blind community have a sense of hearing so acute that they are able to 'hear the very beating of his heart' at a distance ([1914] 1997:15). He finds this extraordinary acuity both mysterious and disturbing. With their stethoscopes doctors acquired an ability to hear with similarly uncanny penetration. The stethoscope unnerved patients by the seemingly magical powers that it lent to the physician (Reiser 1997:831). Indeed, Mol suggests that even for today's patients, the stethoscope represents a 'pretty impressive' technology (2002:61).

While the stethoscope enabled access to a body of sounds for the physician it also created an area of silence for patients: 'What the doctor heard, after all, was not generally discernible to the patient' (Reiser 1997:831). Earlier it was suggested that the stethoscope served to create distance between the doctor and the patient. This distance served the interests of hygiene (though this was not a well-developed concept in Laennec's day, as germs and bacteria had yet to be discovered), of propriety (providing distance between the doctor and female patients) and of perception (creating objective distance for the physician). But the stethoscope had also created a distance of authority and status between doctor and patient. Doctors' 'exquisite sensory training' in auscultation endowed them with specialist expertise (Reiser 1978:94). They were able to 'hear the body in ways inaccessible to lay people' (Sterne

2003b:214). The bodies of doctors came to be reconfigured as repositories of powerful auditory knowledge. Recognized as being possessed of valuable specialist abilities, medical men were accorded an elevated social status (Reiser 1978:94). Auscultation contributed to the creation of a new self-consciousness in doctors, an awareness of their potential to be skilled, knowledgeable and hence respected professionals. It might be argued that through the invention of the stethoscope, a particular kind of doctor was also invented.

Acoustic illumination

As indicated above, Foucault recognizes that the concept of the medical gaze encompasses more than is suggested by the word 'gaze' alone, and should be regarded as 'pluri-sensorial' (1973:165). He notes the importance of listening and touching in the production of medical knowledge and even goes as far as to envisage Laennec listening to a patient's chest (ibid.). But Foucault maintains that in listening with the stethoscope, Laennec is still haunted by a diagnostic image that he is attempting to realize through sound. Listening provides an acoustic illumination of the visually inaccessible space of the bodily interior.

Reiser states that at the time auscultation emerged, physicians were also devising more direct ways to 'visually penetrate the body's opaque skin cover and dark passages' (1978:45). He suggests that the development of the opthalmoscope and laryngoscope, and later of devices for illuminating the vagina, bladder, rectum and stomach, meant that in the latter half of the nineteenth century, vision 'competed with sound as the doctor's main probe of the human interior' (ibid.:55). I discuss the sensory logic underpinning this sensory transition in more detail later, and also consider further ways in which visual technologies presented challenges to the use and value of auscultation in some Western medical settings. In the hospitals in which I conducted my fieldwork, however, sound and listening continued to play a role in the production of medical knowledge about the body. Auscultation and percussion were still in routine use by doctors. Also, as indicated in the previous chapter, a degree of skilled listening was required of some medical professionals in their use of Doppler echocardiography. Indeed, medical applications of ultrasound technology could be construed as a further means by which sound (albeit ultrasound) is used to visualize the bodily interior. In addition, nurses were obliged to employ monitory listening in their work, which necessitated their being attuned to tones from electrocardiograph machines. Monitory listening, however, is arguably not highly skilled and is rarely of critical diagnostic importance, meaning that it is not assigned high value by medical practitioners. Perhaps electrocardiography represents the beginning of a wider shift in medical practice whereby sound and listening will gradually be less and less involved in (high skill and high status) diagnostic practice and will increasingly be directed towards the (lower skill and lower status) monitoring of data presented through auditory display.

Clearly, expertise in auscultation no longer represents the pinnacle of modern medical professionalism and technologies have emerged which offer considerably greater diagnostic power than the stethoscope. But while sound and listening may not be dominant in diagnostic practice in the way they were in the nineteenth and early twentieth centuries, and while, as we will see, their use may even be under threat in some clinical contexts, it is clear that the history of diagnostic listening I have given here is only part of what is, for the time being at least, an ongoing narrative around the acoustic illumination of the body's organs and processes in Western medicine. The sonic mediation of information about bodily spaces, surfaces, states and events continues.

This chapter draws upon material from Tom Rice, 'Sounding Bodies: medical students and the acquisition of stethoscopic perspectives' in *The Oxford Handbook of Sound Studies*, edited by Trevor Pinch and Karin Bijsterveld 2012. By permission of Oxford University Press.

CHAPTER 4

'The Hallmark of a Doctor'

The Stethoscope and the Making of Medical Identity

As the fact that young doctors travelled to Paris to learn auscultation from Laennec illustrates, the hospital in early nineteenth century France was both a place for the housing of the sick poor and one in which doctors and students of medicine received practical training and gained clinical experience (Foucault 1973:64–85). Many hospitals in contemporary Britain continue to function partly as sites of medical education. This was true of both the hospitals in which I conducted fieldwork. At St Thomas' in particular, medical training was a clearly visible facet of the hospital. Medical students could be seen almost every day on the corridors, following the teaching doctors or hanging around waiting for them to turn up, socializing in the café or using the library and computer clusters which were themselves a marker of the hospital's educational purpose.

The students with whom I conducted the majority of my participant observation were in their third year of medical school, and had been asked to ensure they brought stethoscopes of their own to their teaching sessions at St Thomas'. I noticed that considerable excitement and pride surrounded their purchasing of these instruments. The students talked about their stethoscopes a great deal and visibly enjoyed wearing and displaying them. But why did the ownership of a stethoscope carry such significance for the students? Why was the instrument so fundamental to the construction and performance of medical identity, to 'being a doctor', for them?

Kirsch writes that: '[n]o instrument is more closely linked to the medical profession that the stethoscope' (1998). Indeed, so integral to the medical persona has the stethoscope become that doctors are sometimes referred to as 'stethoscopes', in the same way that policemen might be referred to as 'uniforms' or businessmen as 'suits', thus placing in question the very distinction between person and object. Walking down the main corridor of St Thomas', dozens of stethoscopes (in both the literal and the metonymical sense of the term) would move past me. The stethoscope has a high profile in popular as well as medical culture. In the media, images of the instrument are frequently employed to establish the medical nature of services and merchandise. Stethoscopes reach out of adverts, are shown curled around products and are woven into logos. Worn by an actor on stage or screen, the stethoscope immediately establishes that the character is a doctor. Of course, the stethoscope is used in these contexts because it is typically worn by doctors and other medical professionals in 'real life'. But what is it that the stethoscope captures or articulates exactly? How have the material specificities and affordances of this object allowed it to become so symbolically powerful? How have they allowed it to define the clinical role?

Sinclair (1997), himself a qualified doctor-turned-anthropologist, presents a study of medical training based on fieldwork conducted among students at London's University College Hospital where he himself studied. Sinclair's work is firmly grounded in Bourdieu (1980), and he suggests that, through their institutional training, students learn or adopt sets of 'dispositions', which structure the way in which doctors think and act (ibid.:54). Internalizing these dispositions the students take on (both consciously and unconsciously) a doctorly way of being, a doctor 'habitus' (ibid.:60). Indeed, for Sinclair, the primary purpose of medical school is to instil and consolidate the medical habitus within its students.

This chapter argues that in the act of applying the stethoscope as part of a clinical examination, a doctor produces a particularly neat encapsulation or performance of the primary dispositions of the medical habitus described by Sinclair. In their own carrying, handling and use of the stethoscope, medical students are able to move closer to or momentarily realize and fulfil the medical habitus to which they aspire and which they see enacted by teaching doctors and other professional role models around them. The chapter, then, shows how auscultation can be understood as a practice around which wider embodied habits of 'doctorly' thought, action and self-perception are organized. While I have previously pointed to the role of listening in the formation of patient selves, here the use of the stethoscope is shown to be involved in the formation of doctor selves.

The stethoscope can be understood to play an active role in enabling both doctors and medical students to perform and project their medical skill, experience and competence. Though the notion that an inanimate object of any kind might 'play an active role' in any social process or interaction at first seems nonsensical, several authors assert that objects can meaningfully be considered to channel, hold and exert 'agency', a capacity to initiate or participate in social interactions and social life (e.g. Latour 1999, Miller 2005). Focusing on artworks, Gell (1998) suggests that these objects can be understood to have agency in, for instance, the way that they motivate or provoke responses and interpretations from viewers. At the same time, they may act as agents in referencing an artist's skill, thought process, or some other aspect of his or her creativity. Drawing on Gell, this chapter argues that the stethoscope can be understood to hold 'agency', or 'agencies' in the way that it indexes the medical competencies both of individual user/owners and of members of the medical profession more widely. At the same time, through owning different designs of stethoscope and handling them in different ways, doctors and medical students become able to mark their relative status within the hospital hierarchy. The instrument might therefore be understood to have agency in the way that it enables doctors to articulate and express their relative positions within the social structure of the hospital. The chapter points to the mutual mediation of subject and object, doctor (or medical student) and stethoscope that occurs within the hospital. In doing so it builds on Sinclair's discussion of medical training by highlighting the importance of the stethoscope, and by implication, medical instruments and objects more generally, in the formation and mediation of the doctor habitus.

'The hallmark of a doctor'

As indicated above, prior to beginning their first year of 'clinics', the students whose classes I attended during fieldwork had all been asked to acquire a stethoscope. I accompanied some of them to the shops where they made these purchases. It was exciting to slide the lid off the box and see the stethoscope stretched out in its foam inlay like a musical instrument. The metallic shine of the earpieces was hypnotic; the smooth coating of the plastic tubes pleasing to the touch. 'Who could resist the invitation of those dainty headphones?' asks Kracauer. 'They gleam...and entwine themselves around heads all by themselves' (1995:333). Kracauer is writing on early radio use. He describes the manner in which users are seduced by the pleasing design of the technology. The new stethoscopes, too, exercised a peculiar power of attraction.

The students knew that they were to undergo training, becoming familiar with the techniques of auditory focus and sonic differentiation that auscultation requires, but they engaged immediately with their stethoscopes as powerful symbols of their intended profession. They wore them ostentatiously around their shoulders as they paraded down hospital corridors, polishing the diaphragms proudly whilst they stood around chatting. Before entering wards they made careful adjustments to ensure that the ends of their stethoscopes were hanging down evenly from around their necks.

Sinclair remarks in his study that 'the general public's appetite for both written and televised fictional and documentary portrayals of medical life seems insatiable' (1997:5). He also comments on medical students' and junior doctors' avid consumption of such programmes (ibid.). Hospital dramas, in particular *Casualty* and *ER*, were also immensely popular amongst the medical students with whom I conducted research. I was told that these programmes had inspired many students to study medicine in the first place, and that characters in the series now provided professional role models. When I asked members of the firm why they took such pride in their stethoscopes, one of the responses I received was that a doctor wearing a stethoscope was 'such an image from TV'. The characters they admired in programmes such as *ER* were shown carrying stethoscopes. The students liked the idea of being able to reproduce 'the look of the doctor' and having a stethoscope at least brought them closer to being able to do this.

On my very first day of fieldwork, Dr Coltart surprised us all (the firm of students and myself) by explaining that we ourselves were to make an appearance on national television. *City Hospital* was a reality TV show that was filmed inside St Thomas'. The programme followed human-interest stories, with presenters speaking to patients and the staff involved in their treatment. On this occasion the producers wanted some footage of students setting out on the path to becoming doctors and were keen to film a group just starting clinics. They had approached Dr Coltart to see if it would be possible to film his students and he had readily agreed, thinking that it would be an exciting way for us to begin our year.

The stethoscope was to be the focus of the piece. It was felt this would be apt as the students had just bought theirs and so had just acquired the definitive emblem of the profession to which they aspired. The production team would film part of a class on a ward where, supervised by Dr Coltart, the students would examine an elderly female patient. The idea was that the presenter would chat to the patient first and then call the class over and talk to us. Dr Coltart would ask one of us to listen to the patient's heart while another student gave an account of the stethoscope's invention. After a diagnosis had been reached the presenter would finish the piece with words to the effect of 'Well, it's good to see the next generation of doctors progressing so nicely'. There would then be a cut to a different story.

It took some time to decide who would do the listening for the camera but eventually Sue Ann agreed. As none of us had ever studied cardiology before, no one would be able to make an actual diagnosis, so Dr Coltart told Sue Ann to say that she could hear the murmur of mitral regurgitation after she had pretended to listen. Tom, perhaps the most confident student in the group, agreed to give a brief history of the stethoscope, which he had learned during his pre-clinical studies. We were ushered upstairs to the ward where an elderly lady was sitting up expectantly in bed. Cameramen were moving around choosing shots. Then the presenter arrived, former *EastEnders* actress Nadia Sawalha. She checked that Sue Ann and Tom were ready and all of a sudden there were lights and cameras pointing at us and we were on. The following is a transcript of what was televised that morning, reproduced with permission:

Nadia (to the camera): Look! Nine medical students! Their very first day on the ward! (She walks over with the camera following her). Hello! Now, one of you is going to be diagnosing my Mary over there, aren't you?

Sue Ann: Me.

Nadia: First day and on the telly! How good is that? See you in a minute! (She walks over to Mary's bed with the camera following and sits down beside her). Hi Mary! Do you know that that lot (pointing at the students) have got to come over and say what's wrong with you? So, tell me, what is wrong with you?

Mary: I've got left ventricular heart failure and mitral valve regurgitation.

Nadia: So you've basically got to have a...

Mary: Triple heart bypass, which is next Thursday.

Nadia: Did it run in your family, then, the heart problems?

Mary: Yes it did. My dad died of a heart attack at sixty-one and my mum was found dead in bed aged forty-four.

Nadia: You were only a wee thing yourself?

Mary: Aged fourteen.

Nadia: You're also a nurse, aren't you?

Mary: Yes.

Nadia: Does that make it more nerve-wracking being in hospital?

Mary: Not a bit of it.

Nadia: Okay, well look, here they come!

(Dr Coltart arrives with the students and myself following).

Dr Coltart: Hello Mary.

Mary: Hello Dr Coltart.

Dr Coltart: Here's the new crew of students. Bright looking lot, aren't they? I want Sue Ann to have a listen in to see if she can pick up a diagnosis with her stethoscope – you know all about that. So, on you go, Sue Ann. You see, as new medical students they've all got their brand new stethoscopes. This is like the hallmark of a doctor – you've got the stethoscope.

Nadia: Was that really exciting this morning, putting that around your neck? (Students nod). Ah...cool.

Dr Coltart: I've asked Tom over here to tell us briefly how it was invented. When you ask a student who invented the stethoscope you don't expect the answer to come back as Mr Steth. There's a lot more history to it. Tom, tell us, what did you find out?

Tom: It was Rene Laennec in 1816. He was working at the Necker Hospital in Paris and was walking down the street when he saw some street urchins scratching pins on a log. He suddenly realized you could listen to someone's chest through a piece of wood like that because of the resonance. So he rolled up some paper like a log and listened with it, making a monaural stethoscope.

Nadia: Okay, so have we been able to get a diagnosis, Sue, through your rather marvellous stethoscope?

Sue Ann: Well, it sounds like a mild mitral regurgitation.

Nadia: Oh! Is that what she's got?

Dr Coltart: She has, she's got a little leak of the mitral valve and if the heart muscle picks up next week when she has this triple bypass then that should go away, so you've heard it for the last time maybe!

Nadia: Well done, guys! I hope you enjoy your first day. Thank you for letting us be a part of it!

While the medical students are introduced in their own right as the presenter passes on her way to Mary's bed and again as they approach her bedside with Dr Coltart, they are otherwise only presented through the stethoscope and the stethoscope through the medical students. The people and the object are engaged in a kind of mutual performance. There is also a clear sense that the stethoscope represents a kind of trophy. 'Was that really exciting this morning, putting that around your neck?' asks the presenter as if the stethoscope was a medal and should be worn with a pride consistent with that analogy by those who have 'won' it. The students obligingly all nod, smiling, seemingly confirming that wearing a stethoscope does indeed represent, for them, a kind of award. At the same time, Dr Coltart suggests that being able to wear the stethoscope represents a progression into the world of doctors and that the students have now acquired the right to wear the doctor's definitive symbol. The piece, then, reaffirms the centrality of the stethoscope to medical identity, both for the students and for the watching public.

The stethoscope and the doctor habitus

Speaking about wearing his stethoscope, Tom (the student who gave an account of the instrument's invention) said:

> I love wearing it, I love wearing it…I get this feeling when I get into the lift and I've got my stethoscope on and I've been in the hospital all day and I'm feeling rough and I'm feeling tired. I feel like all the other people in the lift should be nice to me, because the stethoscope shows I'm a medical student. I've been walking around the wards all day dealing with people. I feel something like, not superiority, but 'I know what's going on and you guys don't'.

For him, wearing a stethoscope captures the essence of being a medic. He feels like an insider to the dramas unfolding at the hospital. He is busy, working hard for the good of others, exercising knowledge that is denied to or beyond those who do not work in the hospital but are simply passing through it. He is dealing with important problems and should be granted, he feels, respect in the eyes of the public.

In *The Logic of Practice*, Bourdieu discusses the concept of 'habitus', which he suggests 'could be regarded as a subjective but non-individual system of internalised structures, common schemes of perception, conception and action' (1980:60). Habitus is the realization and reproduction of a particular set of 'dispositions', attitudes that determine the practical and ideological approach which a group, and the individuals within that group, take towards reality (ibid.:54). Sinclair (1997) draws heavily on the notion of habitus in his analysis of medical training. He argues that medical school represents a process of inculcation through which the medical habitus is reproduced in new generations of doctors. He points to distinct dispositions that have developed through history, structuring the communal understandings through which doctors think and act. The purpose of medical school is to develop these dispositions within its students. The key dispositions Sinclair identifies are 'Knowledge', 'Experience' and 'Responsibility'. Two other dispositions relevant to the present discussion are 'Idealism' and 'Status'.

Sinclair writes extensively on the origins of the above dispositions and I offer a summary here (ibid.:39–71). As described in the previous chapter, during the anatomical turn in medicine the dissection of corpses became fundamental to the production of medical knowledge. Sinclair suggests, though, that dissection created two related but distinct forms of knowledge. Firstly there was knowledge that was communally visible and accessible, obtained by observation of the dissected body or the study of pictorial or textual representations of it. Secondly, there was knowledge gained through the actual process of dissecting the corpse, which required practical application and skill. For Sinclair the above distinction remains valid in relation to contemporary medical work. He differentiates between Knowledge, which refers to factual learning and to the body of information of which medical students must acquire a grasp, and Experience, which refers to a familiarity with medical cases and an embodied knowledge of how to act in relation to them. Knowledge is gained chiefly through lectures and the study of texts, while Experience is gained through seeing and dealing with patients on the wards. Students must acquire and learn to value these dispositions during their medical training, while qualified doctors should be seen to be in possession of them both.

For Sinclair, anatomy 'was the basis not only for understanding physiology but, increasingly, also for the practice of surgery' (ibid.:50). He suggests that as a result of the prevalence of dissection, the surgeon in the early nineteenth century had a better command of the distinction between normal and abnormal physiology than had his predecessors and a better range of surgical instruments at his disposal. Fewer patients died during operations and successful outcomes increased. Where patients did die they could be quickly dissected, allowing surgeons opportunities to learn from their mistakes. The surgeon's position of being personally able to undertake action that was directed towards achieving beneficial outcomes for the patient leads Sinclair to identify the disposition of Responsibility. Once again, he suggests, this disposition is clearly evident in medical work today. It is 'a desirable attribute, archetypally found in the surgeon holding his patient's life in his hands, and gained by having patients and doing medical things to them' (ibid.:17–8). Responsibility is not unique to surgeons but is found to some extent in all medical actions in which the doctor acts on the patient's behalf and is accountable for that action. Of course, medical students can only accumulate Responsibility gradually as they progress in their careers, but they should show themselves willing to assume it during their training.

Knowledge, Experience and Responsibility are considered by Sinclair to be the most important dispositions within medical practice. However, he also links the improved surgical activities made possible largely through the increasing depth and sophistication of anatomical knowledge (but also advances in antisepsis and anaesthesia) to the disposition of Idealism. While medical practice might, since its inception, have been loosely orientated towards 'doing good' for patients, advances in surgery in particular meant that the potential for medical men to intervene in patients' lives to positive effect became increasingly marked and demonstrable. The disposition of Idealism had growing relevance in a medical sphere in which doctors had growing power to change patients' lives for the better. Sinclair indicates that in medical practice today, Idealism can be understood as the quality of wanting to help people and act in their best interest. Medical students are expected to exhibit this disposition even prior to admission, in their interviews for medical school.

Sinclair connects the disposition of Status to the increasing professionalization of medicine that occurred over the first half of the nineteenth century and which was fully established by the Medical Act of 1858. He points out that the profession had been made credible through the scientific basis of its knowledge that in turn had its origins in the practices of dissection and anatomy. The status of the medical profession continued to grow as a consequence of the increasing value of its knowledge and the effectiveness of its practices, and Sinclair notes that today the medical profession is held in particularly high regard. As a disposition, Status refers to a level of respect that should be accorded to the doctor by his patients, colleagues and society as a whole. Again, this is a disposition which medical students attain partly through qualification, but which is also gradually acquired during their training and progression through professional life.

Of course, unless they happen to be familiar with the work of Sinclair and/or Bourdieu, medical students are not familiar with the concept of habitus or with the notion that in studying medicine they are internalizing a set of dispositions. I would suggest, however, that they are seeking to realize a concept of 'doctorliness', a particular 'way of being' which they consider to be appropriate to or representative of a doctor. I believe it is the fulfilment or realization of this 'doctorly' way of thinking and acting that motivates Tom's deep enjoyment of wearing his stethoscope in the lift. He feels he exhibits Responsibility by working with patients on the wards, or 'dealing with people'. He shows something of both his Experience and Idealism in being able to assist those who need his help. He commands Knowledge of the hospital and its occupants that those around him do not and consequently feels himself to have earned prestige, or Status. If we look closely, what Tom accomplishes is the momentary encapsulation and crystallization of the key dispositions making up the habitus which medical school has taught him to emulate. Importantly, the stethoscope plays a key role in allowing Tom to affirm and articulate his 'doctorliness', communicating it to the other occupants of the lift.

We might conceptualize the stethoscope as a kind of prosthesis. It is an excorporation of the doctor's sense of hearing, a material manifestation of auditory attention. The instrument both compensates for inadequacy in and extends the reach of the doctor's acoustic capacities, increasing his or her power to make observations and diagnostic decisions. The doctor's use of the stethoscope in auscultation arguably produces another cyborg, a fusion of body/organism and machine/technology (Haraway 1991). Alternatively, following Latour, it might be suggested that in everyday medical practice the doctor 'enlists' the stethoscope in order to listen to hearts (1999:178). A 'collective' of human actor and a non-human 'actant' is thereby created (ibid.:174, 180). The ability to hear subtle heart sounds is 'allowed, authorized, enabled, afforded' by the doctor in collaboration with the stethoscope (ibid.:182). By this rationale, both doctor and stethoscope must be understood as participants in auscultation. The power or capacity to act (and in this case, listen) effectively cannot be assigned to the doctor alone. Agency is distributed between both person and thing, doctor and stethoscope.

Like Latour, Gell (1998) also gives consideration to the agency of objects, which he suggests act as extensions of the person. He uses the example of land mines (though any other weapon could be substituted) arguing that these are not simply tools that a soldier uses. Instead, they are things that extend the soldier's capacity to act and initiate events in the war zone: his agency (ibid.:20). Although not agents to the same degree as the soldier, the mines themselves can be considered to possess a degree of agency, as without them the soldier will not be able to realize fully his soldierly aims and intentions (ibid.). Gell goes on to consider artworks, which, he suggests, enable the artist to convey or project his or her creativity into the world, thereby engaging and affecting other people. Artworks, then, also have agency, this time as 'indexes' of the artist's talent or creative power (ibid.:24). In its use as a diagnostic device, the stethoscope might be understood to have agency in a similar way to the soldier's mines. It extends the doctor's sensory capacities and capabilities, allowing him or her the fullest exercise of clinical perception and judgment. But this is not the way, or not the only way, in which Tom uses the instrument in the instance described above. In enacting and projecting his desired identity – that of a medical student well on the way to being a doctor – he also harnesses the stethoscope's agency as an 'index' of the medical profession and the powerful patterns of thought and action through which its members work.

Pretending to doctor status

Many of the students enjoyed their freedom to wear the stethoscope; they took satisfaction from the way that it enabled them to 'play the doctor'. However, a small minority felt flaunting the stethoscope to be something of a cliché and were not keen to parade their new possessions. One of the third year medics to whom I spoke said that if he wore his stethoscope across his shoulders he felt 'like a pretender, a bit of a ponce'. Though he owned a stethoscope he felt he 'knew nothing', and by wearing it was boasting of a skill which he did not actually command. He might have a stethoscope of his own, but he had 'no mastery over it'. Sue Ann felt that although medical students could carry a stethoscope from the third year of their training, they should not wear it until they had actually qualified (usually after five years). Until that time, she said, the stethoscope 'belonged in the pocket' rather than round the neck and that was how she chose to carry hers. Unlike most of her contemporaries, she did not want to pretend to doctor status.

Within the hospital, then, the conspicuous display of the stethoscope could be understood to advertise 'new medical student' status. Third year medical students occupy a low position in the social hierarchy of the hospital. They carry less authority than students in their fourth and fifth years; their lack of qualifications means they are also of lower status than other medical staff, for instance nurses and physiotherapists. Though third year medical students used the stethoscope to differentiate themselves from patients and non-medical staff, and hoped to emphasize their aspiration to become qualified doctors, for those familiar with the professional hierarchy of the hospital their over-enthusiastic exhibition of the stethoscope only served to confirm them in their neophyte position.

Marks writes that: '[t]he stethoscope is the doctor's symbol of office' (1972:16). But of course, at St Thomas' some doctors did not overtly 'wear' their stethoscopes, either from personal preference or because it was not common practice for members of their particular area of expertise to do so. Cardiologists almost invariably carried stethoscopes, but doctors from for instance, psychiatry, psychology and ophthalmology often did not. Also, doctors and medical students were not the only people who carried stethoscopes within the hospital. Nurses sometimes had them, as, for instance, did physiotherapists. Consultant Nurse Elaine Coady, who was based in the Cardiothoracic Unit told me:

> I work as a nurse in a clinic, but I don't wear a uniform, and I have a stethoscope. Now, patients in the heart failure clinic I see time and time again, they get used to the idea that I'm a nurse and I examine their chest and other things, but patients in the chest pain clinic who I only ever see once... I always introduce myself as a nurse. 'I'm Elaine, I'm the *nurse*,' and I emphasize the word and I say 'Your *doctor* has asked me to see you.' Now what I see a lot of them doing is looking at my badge throughout the consultation, so you'll be chatting to them and their eyes kind of go like this...(stares at my ID badge) and you can guarantee that eighty to ninety percent of the time, when you say goodbye to them they say 'Goodbye, doctor.' And I think it's the imagery of not wearing a uniform, having a stethoscope, listening to the chest, listening to heart sounds that conjures up an image... I think that if I was wearing a uniform they wouldn't be saying 'Goodbye, doctor.'

Medical students were also asked to follow the smart-casual dress code and did not wear uniforms. Adopting this style of dress (sometimes with a white coat), like carrying and handling the stethoscope, was part of their integration into and reproduction of the doctor habitus. But it also made it very easy for them to imitate, pass themselves off as, or be mistaken for doctors, particularly by members of the public who were not familiar with the subtleties and nuances of clothing, accessories, bearing and gesture as expressions of professional status within the hospital.

I was generally dressed in smart-casual clothes during fieldwork, and when I donned a stethoscope I found that people made a special effort to make way for me in the corridors or the lifts. Sometimes patients or visitors to the hospital would catch my arm in the corridor and say, 'Excuse me, doctor. Could you tell me where to find...?' The stethoscope was also a helpful facilitator for gaining access to the administration floor to leave messages for Dr Coltart. It acted as a passport. The cardiothoracic department had a swipe-card lock on the door, and though I was authorized to go inside, the card with which I had been issued did not work the lock. Doctors would tend to hold the door open if I was carrying a stethoscope, whereas otherwise they would make no eye contact and, feigning to be unaware of my presence, allow the door to close.

On one occasion, I was standing with two students in the hospital café, *Tom's 2*, when a woman rushed up to us and said, 'Excuse me, doctors, you have to come quickly, my sister has just passed out in the toilets.' We ran to help. It turned out that two nurses were already on the scene, but the incident served as a loud reminder that it is dangerous to play with the symbolic order of the hospital. Although the two students were allowed to be involved in some medical procedures, and although I would not have been reprimanded for helping a woman who had collapsed in a public place, if a similar incident had occurred on the wards and I had had to announce that I was not, in fact, a doctor whilst dressed as one, there could have been many potentially serious repercussions, not least confusion, a wasting of valuable time, and deep personal embarrassment. From then on I only carried the stethoscope in my pocket. Even from there, however, it enacted its power as a symbol of a valued and respected profession. One day I was in an electronics shop on Tottenham Court Road buying a new microphone for my interviews. I went to find my wallet and pulled out the stethoscope. The man behind the counter noticed, and nodding, made a remark about how good he thought it was that I was a doctor. He gave me a discount of £2.50.

Stethoscope convention

Proficiency in auscultation requires years of practice. Doctors slowly improve their listening skills throughout their training and careers. As a consequence, it tends to be senior doctors who are most expert at auscultation. Their ability to hear quickly and decisively becomes a marker of their seniority. In the same way, a pronounced hierarchy of stethoscope ownership and display was evident at St Thomas'. The stethoscope that a doctor wore seemed to be a

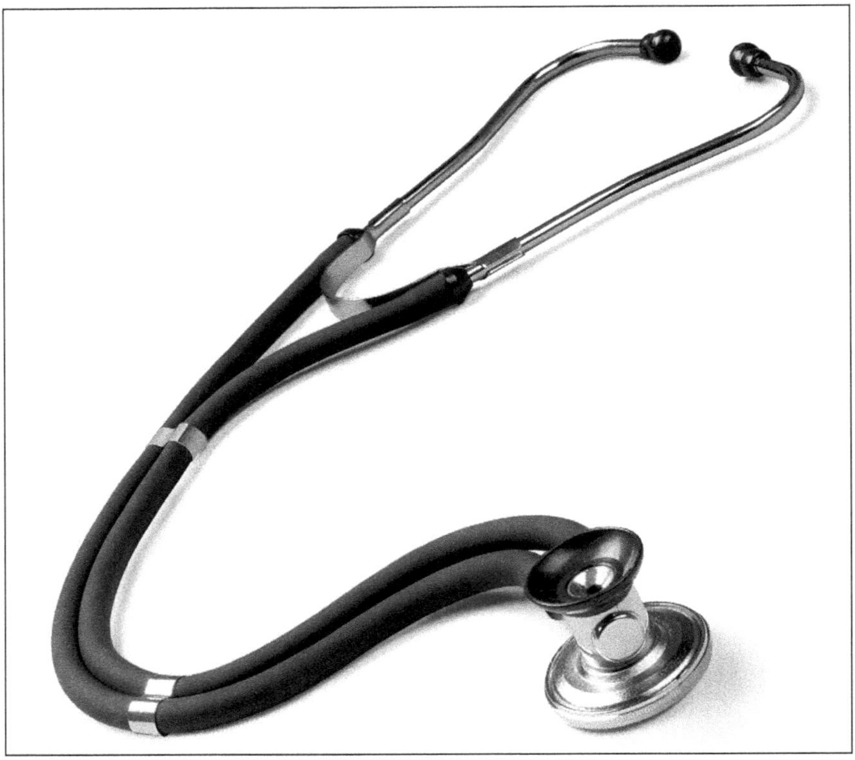

Figure 2 *The Traditional Sprague.*

kind of visual/material representation or manifestation of the knowledge and status he held.

Prior to their introduction to auscultation, the students were given little advice on what kind of stethoscope to buy. All those in the rotation with which I was working purchased a Littman Classic II SE with black tubing. Wanting to fit in, I thought I would buy the same. At the shop, however, I found that the tubing came in hunter green, navy blue, Caribbean blue, black, burgundy or orange. Having been assured there was no colour code (having a red stethoscope, for instance does not signify that you are a nurse, it just goes well with a white uniform) I spent some time deliberating before I chose a navy one, which I thought was only subtly different from the black and looked a bit more stylish.

I did not hold on to my new stethoscope for long, however. A few days later at the end of one of our teaching sessions, Rishi, with whom I was beginning to become friends, asked a little nervously if I wouldn't mind swapping stethoscopes with him. He had an identical twin brother who was also a medical student. They had gone to buy stethoscopes separately on the same day and had each bought the same design with the same colour tubing.

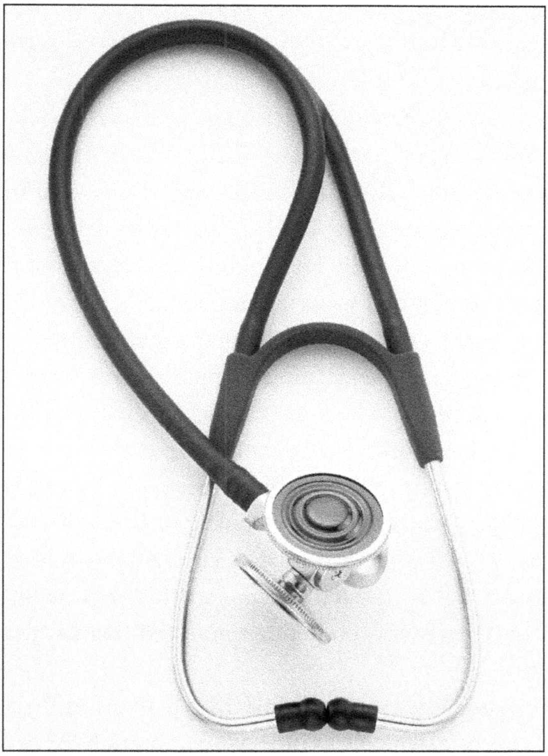

Figure 3 *The Harvey Triple Head.*

Rishi felt it would be an important marker of his individuality if he had a stethoscope that was not the same as his brother's. He wondered whether it might be possible for him to have my stethoscope with its navy blue tubing and for me to take his with its black tubing. In actual fact I had already become quite attached to my navy stethoscope, but I was keen to make friends and thought this exchange might help cement our developing relationship. I said that would be fine, and we did the swap.

As it turned out, a few months later Rishi upgraded his stethoscope to a Littman Cardiology III. This was considered by the other students in the firm to be a bit 'keen' or 'spoddy'. Rishi, though, had never disguised the fact that he was passionate about his studies and the other students seemed to accept this with a minimum of good-humoured teasing. Their ridicule became much more intense, however, when Rishi upgraded again and bought the still more expensive Littman Master. Rishi was now thought by both students and teaching doctors to be acting presumptuously. He risked looking as though he had ideas above his station. Designs like the Cardiology III or the Master tended to be used only by more senior doctors – registrars and consultants. Rishi was laying claim to an object that was properly the symbolic holding of someone much his senior. Having been reminded of this by his peers, Rishi reverted to using the Cardiology III in clinics. He said he would only use the Master to practise listening at home.

Some senior doctors boasted particularly unusual types of stethoscope. One registrar, for instance, owned the Traditional Sprague, in which each earpiece is connected directly to the diaphragm by its own individual tube. A consultant I met used a Harvey Triple Head, which has two diaphragms as well as a bell (the piece, normally forming the reverse side of the diaphragm, which is used for listening to low frequency sounds). It was the tendency for senior doctors to carry unusual models of stethoscope that led to the joke: 'What's oddly shaped and hangs off an anus? A consultant's stethoscope.' Cardiology was considered to be a prestigious specialism within the hospital where I conducted fieldwork. It was thought to attract ambitious and high achieving people and its senior doctors were generally regarded as having large egos. At the same time, most senior positions in cardiology at St Thomas' were, at the time of my fieldwork at least, occupied by men. On two occasions I heard nurses remark that the stethoscopes worn by consultants were phallic extensions and that there was competition amongst them as to whose was the most impressive.

Students on the chest rotation were invited to sit in on a weekly event called the 'echo meeting', which was otherwise only attended by senior doctors working on the Cardiothoracic Unit. The meeting was at eight in the morning and was not compulsory, but was supported by a pharmaceutical company which provided delicious breakfasts of bacon sandwiches and fruit juice, so a larger number of students than might ordinarily be expected would manage to attend. At the meeting a doctor who was an expert in echocardiography would review the cardiac ultrasound scans of cases within the hospital in which findings had proved particularly interesting or unusual. On one morning before a teaching session it emerged that two of the students in the firm had been to the echo meeting earlier in the day while the rest of us had missed it. The two who had attended were quizzed by their colleagues: Had anything interesting been shown? Which of the senior doctors that the firm had encountered had been there? 'They were all there,' said one of the attendees. 'Believe me, it could have been a fucking stethoscope convention.'

Of course, the stethoscope is not only something owned, carried and worn. It is also entangled with the actions and routines of the clinical examination. As a consequence, as was indicated in the previous chapter, the stethoscope is involved in the articulation of the relationship between doctor and patient. During auscultation the patient accepts the doctor placing the stethoscope upon his or her chest. He or she is often obliged to be partially undressed while the doctor is fully clothed, to be passive while the doctor is active, silent whilst the doctor listens and thinks. The patient obeys the doctor's cues to move into particular positions, to take deep breaths and so on. In the stethoscopic examination the doctor's skill, experience, knowledge and status relative to that of the patient become obvious and overt.

But the stethoscope is also involved in the expression of more subtle dynamics of the doctor-patient interaction. Observing Dr Coltart during his consultations, I noticed that he tended to use his stethoscope rather like a conductor's baton. When listening to a patient explaining a problem he would sit holding the tube of the instrument in his right hand, tapping the diaphragm slowly and meditatively, as if thinking. When he thought the time had come to examine the patient he would point to the couch with it. While listening he would move the stethoscope around with remarkable fluency, pressing the diaphragm to the appropriate points on the chest and listening with brief, intensely focused moments of concentration. Having listened he would usually return to his chair and hold the diaphragm in his hand, cupping it in his palm as he explained what he thought should be done. When he felt it was time for movement he would stand up, letting the stethoscope drop, swinging and dangling from around his neck, creating movement that echoed his sudden animation. Here, it seems, 'mind, body and tool are on very intimate terms' (Haraway 1991:65).

Dr Coltart's deft use of the stethoscope was derived from his frequent use of the instrument over more than thirty-five years and his close familiarity with the progression of the clinical examination. His particular way of handling the stethoscope constituted a performance of skill, knowledge and confidence in the clinical interaction that was taking place. Above I suggested that the medical student named Tom used the stethoscope in creating a demeanour of clinical proficiency. Dr Coltart is arguably employing the instrument in a similar way, drawing on its power to confer an aura of medical authority. But Dr Coltart's actions also reveal the stethoscope's capacity to mediate his more individual or particular qualities as a doctor. It allows him to articulate his deftness and confidence, serving as a sensitive conduit of his skill; the stethoscope allows him to express the minutiae of his clinical persona.

For other doctors to whom I spoke, too, the stethoscope seemed to be essential to the realization of their professional identities. 'I would be lost without a stethoscope. I wouldn't feel complete,' one doctor commented when I asked him what would happen if he found himself at work without one. He continued:

> If I forget it at home I try to find one when I get to the hospital and carry it around with me, but I would consider being late for work rather than

> coming in without my stethoscope. If I get to the corner and realize I have forgotten it, I will certainly go back for it. If I get to the tube station and realize I've forgotten it, I will hesitate for a minute, and then go back for it.

These remarks convey a sense of the doctor's close connection to the stethoscope, built up through repeated use over a number of years. But they also provide an illustration and elaboration of the particular agencies ascribed to the instrument. It can be understood to have agency in the way that it enables the doctor to exercise his full diagnostic capability. At the same, though, it is integral both to the realization of a generalized medical habitus, and to deep, intensely personal feelings of professional competency and completeness.

Stethoscopes as (auto)biographical objects

One day during fieldwork the medical students with whom I was working were talking about their stethoscopes. Diane said that it was exciting to know that this instrument was one you could expect to have with you throughout your medical career. Rishi justified the money his Littman Cardiology III had cost by saying he would be using the same instrument for a very long time to come. The stethoscope is felt to be a tool that will be present at and used in a huge number of interactions; it is an object around which memories or associations can be concentrated and organized – what Hoskins (1998) describes as a 'biographical object'. Students quickly became habituated and attached to their own stethoscopes, often remarking that they were only able to hear properly with these. There seemed to be a strong sense of individual ownership and a general dislike of swapping, lending or borrowing these particular instruments. Having bought a stethoscope it was possible to pay extra to have it engraved with one's name or initials, but none of the students I met had chosen to do this. When I discussed the service with Tom and Diane, they each agreed that their stethoscopes were already distinctively their own, despite the objects being of the same design and colour and seemingly identical.

In an article entitled 'On Being a Doctor: what the stethoscope said', Salomon (2001) describes her feelings of attachment to a stethoscope which is now broken and must be replaced. She writes:

> You might think it overly sentimental to care about a fifteen-year-old stethoscope, now broken, a dud…My stethoscope has come to the end of the line, so to speak, lived out its life expectancy perhaps, and no longer works. It's time to get a new one. So why the fuss? (ibid.:56)

She goes on to explain that her stethoscope has accompanied her throughout her medical career, touching nearly every one of the hundreds of patients she has examined. Her stethoscope is a storied instrument, 'often bloodied during resuscitations' (ibid.). It has absorbed or been inscribed with the events in which it was involved. 'If this stethoscope could speak,' she writes, 'it would tell stories of all my patients' (ibid.).

Ultimately, of course, Salomon is throwing her stethoscope away. Though she has formed an emotional attachment with the object, she will no doubt quickly replace it with another. Stethoscopes, after all, are mass-produced, disposable and can be easily substituted. Nonetheless, the article indicates how a ubiquitous object can become closely linked to the life of its owner (Miller 2008). For Salomon the stethoscope becomes a reference point for the various demands and challenges she has met in her work. It is an object around which a particular personal history is organized, and a sense of self developed through a fifteen-year career in medicine is defined. In a similar way, a registrar to whom I spoke told me about a charity that collected unwanted or obsolete medical equipment from UK hospitals, sending it to third world countries where it might still be useful. Stethoscopes were one of the items they were keen to receive. As a doctor friend of his was working to galvanize interest in the charity and solicit contributions from St Thomas', he had thought he might give his old stethoscope as a donation. He explained, however, that in the end he had found it too hard to separate himself from the instrument that he had used as a medical student and which, he pointed out, he had had with him on the very first day of his career. 'I couldn't give it away in the end,' he said. 'It's too precious to me.'

A junior doctor to whom I spoke during my research told me that his father had also been a doctor and had found it difficult to 'let go' of medicine after his retirement. For years he had carried his stethoscope around with him wherever he went. He would not relinquish it. Eventually one of his children had organized a small ceremony for him to 'pass on' his stethoscope to the doctor now in charge of the practice where he had worked. This formal, physical separation from his stethoscope was deemed necessary in order for him to accept that he no longer practised as a doctor, a profession and a way of being through which he had defined himself throughout his life. Here the stethoscope perhaps becomes what Gonzalez describes as an 'autobiographical object', 'a trace, and a replacement for the intangible aspects of desire, identification and social relations' (Gonzalez 1995:134).

A close personal/professional identification with the stethoscope was also already developing among the third year students with whom I worked. A student to whom Rishi introduced me said she had taken her stethoscope with her when she went away over the Christmas break. She hadn't used it, nor had she intended to, but she had wanted to have it with her. 'I suppose it was because I'm a medical student,' she explained. 'I'm proud to have come this far, and I'm focused on what I want to be.' She said she felt the instrument was 'like a passport.' It identified her, if only in this particular instance to herself, as a future doctor.

Stethoscopes as 'agents,' doctors as 'patients'

At the beginning of this chapter, the stethoscope was identified as the definitive symbol of the doctor in popular culture. The medical students I encountered during fieldwork enjoyed wearing and displaying their new stethoscopes because they recognized the instrument as the icon of their intended profession. This iconic status emerges, I have suggested, through the instrument's mediation of the movements, gestures and attitudes that I align with a medical habitus. It is because using the stethoscope allows the expression of the key dispositions of this habitus, representing their encapsulation, their crystallization, that the instrument has come to be considered emblematic of the medical profession. This chapter, then, underlines the fundamental validity and utility of Sinclair's account of the medical habitus. But it also seeks to build on his discussion by considering the important role played by one particular medical instrument in the formation and articulation of that habitus.

Sinclair is sensitive to the ways in which the materiality of spaces inside the hospital (for instance, the layout of wards) both reflects and reproduces established patterns of social interaction. He suggests, for example, that beds are arranged on the wards in such a way that they allow patients to be effectively encircled by teaching doctors accompanied by groups of medical students (1997:214–18). This spatial organization affords the construction of what Sinclair sees (following Goffman 1997) as essentially theatrical spaces for the performance of medical dispositions (ibid.). The spatial organization of ward environments, Sinclair argues, reflects a preoccupation with performance and theatricality that permeates Western hospital practice and which originated in the anatomy theatre that was designed to enable medical students and other interested parties to observe the dissection of bodies. Sinclair's sensitivity to medical environments and their spatial arrangement, however, does not carry over into a discussion of the involvement of medical instruments in the mediation of dispositions. As this chapter illustrates, medical training in fact creates opportunities for the establishment of intimate connections between objects, persons and practices in the medical environment.

The notion of intimacy between objects and persons is particularly pertinent to the discussion of stethoscope use. We have seen how medical students and professionals can develop close connections, and even affective bonds, with their stethoscopes through using them several times a day often for years on end. They can acquire a detailed embodied knowledge and appreciation of these instruments. At the same time, stethoscopes become intertwined with deeply engrained routines and patterns of action, such as clinical examinations, that constitute an important part of the fabric of many doctors' professional lives. The affordances of the stethoscope extend far beyond the provision of a means of diagnostic listening alone. Auscultation involves a complex set of mutual mediations of person and thing, subject and object.

Gell makes a distinction between 'agents' and 'patients'. '[T]he patient is the object which is causally affected by an agent's action' (1998:22). Patients are the counterparts of agents: objects or channels of their agency. Illustrating this distinction Gell uses the example of a car (ibid.). Ordinarily, as a person drives a car, he or she is in the agent position in relation to the car, which is the patient. If the car breaks down or refuses to start, however, then, even if only momentarily, the positions change. The car takes over not as an intentioned actor, but as initiator of events, actions and responses. The person is in the patient position, while the car is the agent. This chapter has indicated that the stethoscope can be understood to hold different kinds of agency that are harnessed by medical students and doctors as they seek to produce and project their particular clinical identities and relative statuses within the hospital. But some doctors evidently depend on the stethoscope to live out their particular understanding not only of what kind of person a doctor is, but also of what kind of persons they themselves are. Here, then, not only do stethoscopes become agents, but interestingly, doctors are their patients. As we shall see later in the book, however, the instrument has become involved in the narration of professional as well as personal events. Doctors have come to use the stethoscope as a means of reflecting on the life course of the medical profession itself.

This chapter draws on material from Tom Rice (2010) 'The hallmark of the doctor: the stethoscope and the making of medical identity', *Journal of Material Culture* 15(3):287–301, Sage Publications Ltd. Reproduced with permission.

CHAPTER 5

Learning to Listen

Auscultation and the Transmission of Auditory Knowledge

The students with whom I conducted participant observation were embarking on three 'clinical years' involving sessions of supervised contact with patients on the hospital wards. They were to be introduced to the procedures and techniques necessary for their future work as doctors. The students sometimes remarked that while the pre-clinical phase of their education had, broadly speaking, been orientated towards 'brain work', the clinical years would be devoted to 'body work'. In making this essentially Cartesian distinction, students recognized what they perceived to be two different kinds of knowledge that were in the process of transfer in the two educational stages. The classroom/lecture theatre years generally involve the passing on of information – theoretical, factual, and schematic – while the final three years, characterized by 'situated learning' in the clinical setting, are more concerned with the transmission of practical skills (Lave and Wenger 1991). The students were also demonstrating awareness of the fact that while medical work is directed towards the patient's body, it also involves the doctor's body, or in their case, that of the medical student. Competence in diagnosis and in the management and administration of care demands well-honed senses and practised skills. Student bodies must be trained.

The previous chapter introduced Sinclair's work, and suggested that he positions medical school as a process through which the medical habitus, a distinctive set of medically orientated skills and attitudes, is reproduced in new generations of doctors. The use of habitus as a structure may be helpful in conceptualizing medical education in general terms, but there is a danger that the detail and subtleties of the acquisition of specific skills may obscured or overlooked. This chapter aims to reveal some of the sensory complexities of auscultation, a practice which might otherwise tend to be subsumed by, or regarded as merely another technique embedded within, a wider medical habitus. It looks at the ways in which students are taught to focus and concentrate their senses of hearing, and how they learn to differentiate what they at first experience as very similar sounds. At the same time, the chapter challenges a presumed bodily uniformity that is implicit within the habitus concept and which, for instance, allows Sinclair to position medical students as vessels or blanks in and through whom the medical habitus is regenerated. Drawing on the experiences of a medical student with serious hearing difficulties, the chapter provides an example of how schemes of perception are assimilated in diverse ways by those who encounter them. It illustrates the fact that perceptual abilities and aptitudes vary, so that in learning to listen, creativity and resourcefulness are continually demanded of teachers and students alike.

Listening as a 'technique of the body'

The ethnographies of Feld (1996), Gell (1995), and Weiner (1991) are of particular relevance to any discussion of the ways in which listening is learned. These anthropologists each observe and describe complex forms of auditory knowledge and engagement among the Kaluli, Umeda, and Foi respectively. Feld, for instance, illustrates how an understanding of the ways in which Kaluli people engage with the soundscape of their forest habitat (produced by moving water, birdsong, and insects) is crucial for comprehending the nature of their intertwined language, topography, aesthetics and cosmology (Feld 1990; 1991; 1996; 2003). The Kaluli inhabit a steep and rain-forested area, rich in the sounds of running and falling water, insects, birds and other animals. Feld suggests that they respond to the multilayered sonic ecology in which they live through an equally multilayered system of sonic knowing. Kaluli notions of spatiality and emplacement are formed through their largely acoustic negotiation of their physical surroundings, which are so thick with undergrowth that hearing is often more useful than vision, particularly as a distance sense. At the same time, Kaluli language, in relation to place-naming especially, is rich in onomatopoeia and sonic ideophones, echoing sounds in the environment and reflecting the sonic qualities of particular sites. Kaluli also draw on acoustic presences in their music-making and poetry, with birdsong and insects providing melodic themes, textures and musical structures. The cries and songs of birds are in many cases understood to be the voices of ancestors, calling to their human relatives, so that sounds are also closely intertwined with local cosmology and are interpreted in such a way that they provoke distinctive affective responses of longing and loss which Feld considers fundamental to Kaluli sociality (ibid.).

Also working in Papua New Guinea, Gell (1995) has conducted work amongst a group known as the Umeda, who inhabit a landscape much like that of the Kaluli. The forest is sufficiently dense that it is never possible to gain a visual vantage point. Gell describes how, as a visual thinker, he became deeply frustrated by his inability to gain a visual perspective on the village in which he was staying, and was forced to re-assess his ambition to construct the village as a visually discrete entity in his intellectual imagination (ibid.:236). Gell details his gradual realization that 'the balance between vision and other sensory modalities was differently struck where the Umeda were concerned' (ibid.:237). They displayed striking auditory acuity in their engagement with their forest environment, which, for Gell, represented a 'reorganization of sensibility' (ibid.:235). He describes the Umeda as an 'auditory culture' (ibid.:236). In a further ethnographic study, Weiner (1991) describes how the Foi, also of Papua New Guinea, demonstrate an acute awareness of their sonic environment, and possess a sophisticated vocabulary to describe the sounds within it.

All three authors produce fascinating accounts of the importance of sound in the lives of the communities they study, conveying how informants hear their worlds. Feld produces especially evocative passages, describing the distinctive acoustic texture of the Bosavi rainforest (1996:100). He is also proactive in documenting his own processes of learning to listen as an ethnographer, placing the sound-recorder at the centre of his research. He describes how he would play his forest soundscape recordings to his informants, allowing them to twiddle the knobs of the cassette player, creating 'an ethnoaesthetic negotiation' through which he was able to begin to understand how the Kaluli hear 'the dimensionality of forest sound, how they would balance a mix of birds, water, cicadas, voices and so forth' (Feld and Brenneis 2004:467). In a sense, in combination, Feld's writings and recordings offer the reader/listener a lesson in how to hear like a Kaluli.

These 'ethnographies of sound' tell us a great deal about how communities attach salience and meaning to particular sounds and categories of sounds (Gell 1995:233). They show the manner in which sensory knowledge develops through ongoing interaction with the environment. Feld writes that the Kaluli 'way of sensing and hearing the world is internalized as bodily knowledge, part of the everyday 'body hexis' (Bourdieu 1977:8), the naturalized regime of 'body techniques' (Mauss [1935]1979 [1935]) basic to routine Kaluli encounters in their world' (1996:100). There is a lot in this citation, and it deserves further exploration.

Feld draws on Mauss, suggesting that the Kaluli way of hearing the world is part of a naturalized regime of 'body techniques'. In his famous work on techniques of the body, Mauss suggests that skills such as swimming, walking, dancing and running are practised differently from society to society. Growing up, a child learns the particular style of performing these actions practised by those around him or her. Mauss uses the term 'habitus' (later developed by Bourdieu) to describe these culturally specific sets of embodied habits for action, and suggests that the habitus is acquired through usually informal education based on imitation (ibid.:73). Children copy those actions they have seen successfully performed by people in whom they have confidence, or who hold authority over them. In this way, effective means of using the body to achieve goals are passed on through generations and become tradition (ibid.:74–6). Although Feld does not state this, Mauss points out that culturally specific techniques of sensory perception are among those techniques of the body acquired by children at a young age. He writes of the weaned child: '[i]t can eat and drink; it is taught to walk; it is trained in vision, hearing, in a sense of rhythm and form and movement, often for dancing and music...' (ibid.:79). By drawing on Mauss, then, Feld suggests that Kaluli learn and adopt a particular way of engaging with the sounds of their environment from a young age.

Feld also draws on Bourdieu's concept of bodily 'hexis', which is related to that of habitus (1977:87). Bourdieu uses the term 'hexis' to refer to a state in which a particular habitus becomes consolidated and takes on a degree of permanence. Again, although he does not state this explicitly, Feld seems to suggest that we can understand the hexis as encompassing culturally habitual ways of using and directing the senses, including the sense of hearing.

The concepts of habitus and hexis are very useful in an attempt to understand how culturally particular ways of listening and hearing develop and are reproduced across generations. But at the same time, interesting particularities of embodied knowledge may be engulfed or obscured by the 'slackness', or scale of habitus as a concept (Margolis 1999:68). Also, both Mauss and Bourdieu seem to presume a kind of bodily uniformity, implying that the learning of embodied skills proceeds smoothly and almost with inevitability. So although relevant and productive, Feld's use of these theorists obscures a great deal that might be of value to a person interested in the teaching and learning of auditory knowledge. What particular perceptual skills does the 'body hexis' to which he alludes involve, and in exactly what ways is it reproduced among individuals or across generations? Feld's analysis also appears to position shared ways of knowing through sound as apparently unproblematic for the Kaluli, unaffected by differences of perceptual sensitivity or interpretation. It is tempting to ask what issues are presented at an individual and societal level for a person born deaf or hard of hearing into such an 'auditory culture' (Gell 1995:236).

Despite having been described as 'medicine's acoustic culture' (Sterne 2003b:191), it is clear that auscultation does not represent a system of auditory knowledge of the depth or complexity of those described in the ethnographies of Feld, Gell or Weiner. Medical students will not learn to auscultate in the same way that, for instance, Kaluli acquire the 'naturalized regime of "body techniques" that constitute their way of 'sensing and hearing the world' (Feld 1996:100). Yet perhaps because it is encountered in adulthood, and because it situates listening as a conscious act that requires reflection and necessitates attempts at articulation, auscultation might represent a practice in which the dynamics of a kind of auditory skill can be accessed and described closely, rather than being couched in vague terms as 'body techniques'. Cohen (2010) draws attention to the importance of detail in accounts of the making and re-making of knowledge. She describes the potential of ethnographic engagement in communities of practice to reveal the micro-mechanisms and processes underpinning human knowledge. The example of auscultation presents a valuable opportunity to probe the underlying organizational and operational workings of a system of auditory knowledge.

The 'lub dub'

On our first day of the chest rotation I sat with a group of eight medical students around a table in a seminar room. Dr Coltart asked, 'What sound does a heart make?' From our blank expressions it was apparent that none of us knew. This seemed at odds with the fact that most people know what a heart sounds like. As Ackerman points out, '[w]e're used to associating the heart with sound' (1990:190). Even though one might not actually listen to a heart often, one is sometimes aware of one's own heart pumping and the texture of sound that it creates in the ears. The beating heart also has a high profile in popular culture and is often used in television and film soundtracks. But while recognizing the sound might be easy, describing it is evidently more difficult. With no answer forthcoming, Dr Coltart responded to his own question:

> You might be familiar with the song by Peter Sellers and Sophia Loren in which they sing about her heart 'going boom boody-boom'. Well, this describes the heartbeat quite nicely. 'Boom boody-boom' suggests the heartbeat has four components: 'boom', then 'boo-dy', and another 'boom'. In fact the heart does have these four sounds, but because of the way our ears are designed we can't easily separate the many components. So in medicine we say the heart has two main sounds. We say it goes 'lub dub'.

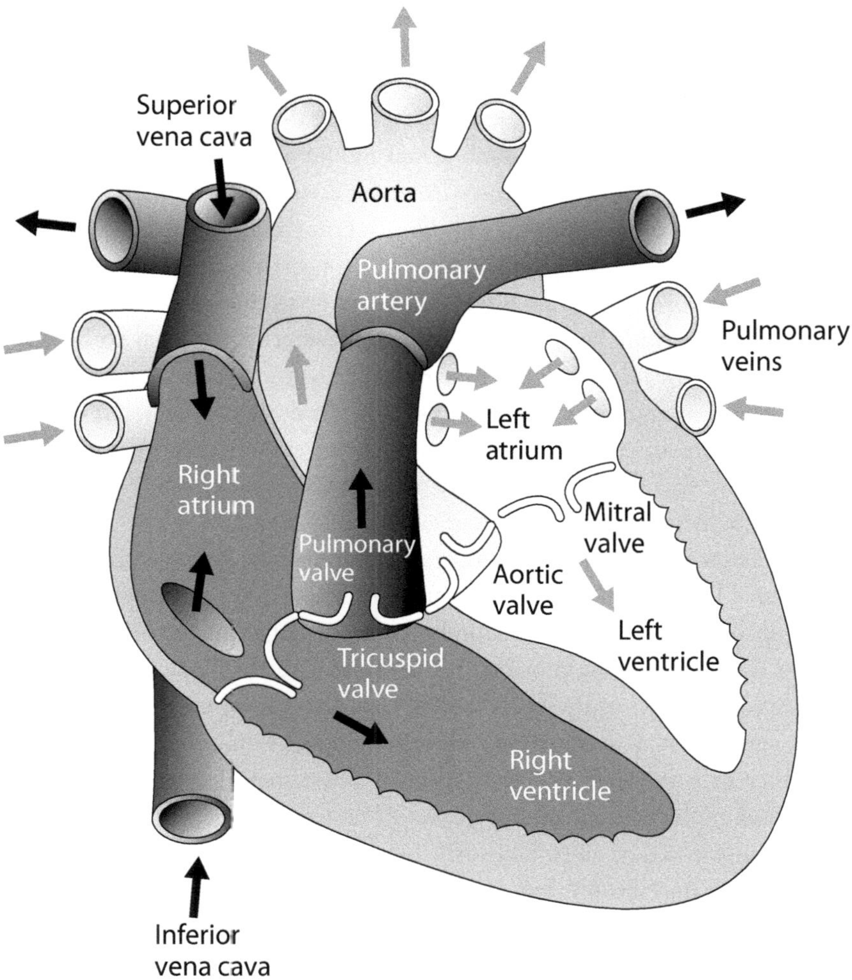

Figure 4 *A simple diagram of the heart. Reproduced with permission of the Texas Heart Institute: http://www.texasheart.org.*

He went on to explain that the first heart sound, the 'lub', is caused by the closure of the mitral and tricuspid valves, and the second, the 'dub', by the closure of the aortic and pulmonary valves. Figure 4, showing the valves and their position in relation to the rest of the heart, may be helpful here.

Normally when blood flows around the heart and across the valves, it does so smoothly, meaning that the only sounds that can be heard through a stethoscope are the closing snaps of the valves, which create the 'lub' and 'dub'. Sometimes, though, a physiological event triggers the blood flow to become turbulent and this turbulence produces what are known as 'heart murmurs'. For instance, if a valve becomes stiff for some reason (e.g. through calcification) and blood is forced through a narrower opening than is normally made by a valve (this restriction of blood flow is known as 'stenosis'), turbulence will be created and a murmur produced. If the valve fails to close properly, or becomes 'floppy', then blood passing through it will flow back (a development known as 'regurgitation') and another murmur will be produced, though at a different stage in the cardiac cycle and with a different sound. Problems with valves are not the only cause of murmurs. Holes in the septum (the muscle wall separating the two sides of the heart), for instance, can cause large volumes of blood to be forced back and forth between the chambers, producing a murmur known as a 'shunt'. Some murmurs appear to have no physiological basis at all, being caused by unexplained turbulence in the blood flow. These are known as 'innocent' or 'flow' murmurs. In general, though, heart murmurs are linked to malfunctioning valves. Dr Coltart claimed that murmurs are the cardiologist's 'bread and butter'. Most of our rotation was therefore devoted to learning to hear and identify them.

In Chapter 1 it was suggested that auscultation is an example of 'listening-in-search' (Truax 2001:22). It is also a type of what Chion describes as 'causal listening', namely 'listening to a sound in order to gather information about its source' (1994:25). Having provided his students with basic oral instruction as to how auscultation of the heart works, Dr Coltart went on to offer further, more sophisticated explanations of how subtleties of pitch, rhythm and dynamics in a murmur express particular physiological changes. In doing so, he communicated an interpretative structure through which a range of heart sounds could be given diagnostic meaning referenced to physical events in the bodily interior. But instructing the students actually to recognize the sounds occurring in patients was more complicated, and required a number of pedagogic strategies.

It is important to point out that auscultation of the heart tends to be used in the context of a more general examination which normally includes the taking of a clinical history, a series of careful observations from the foot of the bed and the taking of pulses as well as many other small checks and procedures, all of which shape the listener's expectations of what will be heard. *The Oxford Handbook of Clinical Medicine* makes this point plain. Its authors claim that auscultation is

> generally, but wrongly, held to be the essence of cardiovascular medicine at the bedside. A caricature of cardiology ward rounds is of the anxious junior gabbling through the history, while noting his chief's fingers twisting his stethoscope, impatient to 'get down to the main business' of listening to the heart – thereby blotting out all talk in favour of a few blissful minutes communing with the 'lub' and the 'dub'. This is absurd ... if you spend time

> listening to the history, and feeling pulses, auscultation should hold few surprises: you will often already know the diagnosis.
>
> (Longmore, Wilkinson and Torok 2001:39)

However, while stethoscopic listening forms just part of a repertoire of diagnostic practices and techniques available to the doctor, at St. Thomas' it was also regarded as an important skill in its own right.

Before listening

With the exception of the initial class in which we were introduced to the theoretical principles of auscultation, sessions for the chest rotation took place on the cardiothoracic wards. Dressed in white coats and clutching notebooks and stethoscopes, we followed Dr Coltart to the bedsides of patients who he judged to be of high 'instructive value' (Foucault 1973:59). This almost invariably meant that they had a heart murmur of some kind. We formed a semi-circle around the bed with Dr Coltart at the head on the patient's immediate left, spatially indexing his status and authority in relation both to his students and to the patient. One of us then pulled the privacy curtain closed.

Dr Coltart emphasized the importance of maintaining good relationships with patients, and in a polite and good-humoured way he introduced us as 'young doctors' to those he had chosen as models or exemplars. He then asked for our observations. Was the patient sitting up? Was he or she speaking comfortably; breathing evenly and regularly; speaking and behaving compliantly? Was the patient over or underweight? Were there scars from previous operations? Were there bandages, tubes or cylinders at the bedside? After gathering answers to his questions, Dr Coltart demonstrated the cardiovascular examination, drawing attention to particular signs of the patient. Among the checks involved were the inspection of the patient's hands and fingers, feeling of pulses in the wrist and neck, noting the colouration of the cornea and health of the teeth, and feeling for any abnormal vibrations through chest palpation.

Having demonstrated these examination stages, Dr Coltart proceeded to the auscultation of the heart. He emphasized that the stethoscope's diaphragm (the part pressed to the patient's chest) should be cleaned with alcohol to prevent the transmission of pathogens and warmed against the back of the hand so it would not feel too cold against the patient's skin. He then showed us how to move our hands over the chest in order to find the 'apex beat', the lowest and outermost point at which the beat of the heart can be felt. This is the point at which cardiac auscultation should begin. Inserting the earpieces of his stethoscope and taking the diaphragm carefully in his hand, Dr Coltart requested that we remain quiet in order to optimize conditions for listening. Doctors, like Ituri pygmies (Turnbull 1961) and Umeda (Gell 1995), preserve a degree of discipline around noise, recognizing the importance of quiet at times when careful listening is necessary. Drawing our attention to the need to push down with the diaphragm so as to make a firm connection with the flesh, Dr Coltart quickly listened at the apex beat, and then indicated how we should move the stethoscope to other 'key points' (see Figure 5) where sounds produced by the heart valves can be most easily discerned. In doing so, he effectively marked out an acoustic topography, a map of listening points on the patient's chest. After the demonstration, Dr Coltart instructed his students to auscultate the patient's heart in turn. They tried hard to imitate Dr Coltart's listening postures and to reproduce the assured air with which he handled the stethoscope. The students found themselves struggling, however, not only with the more overt bodily actions, but also with the subtler perceptual processes of listening.

Non-sense

Using a stethoscope for the first time can be a disconcerting experience. On inserting the earpieces, the sounds to which one is accustomed disappear. The outside world is sealed off; it becomes muted, distant. Scientists working in psychoacoustics have observed that during experiments carried out using headphones, 'physiological noise of vascular origin' (i.e. noise created by the heartbeat and the circulation of blood, also known as 'self-generated noise') becomes trapped inside the ear (Anderson and Whittle 1971; Soderquist and Lindsey 1972). This effect is also produced by the earpieces of the stethoscope so that, paradoxically, the first heart sounds one hears upon inserting them are often one's own. One also quickly learns that the diaphragm of the stethoscope is highly sensitive. The tiniest knock or scrape transmits sudden and painfully loud sounds down the tubes into the ears. After experiencing a few of these unpleasant sonic shocks, one begins to handle the stethoscope with great care.

Placing the stethoscope on the patient's chest can also be perturbing at first because it involves entering the cocoon of warm air that surrounds his or her body. This air is charged with the patient's smell, pleasant or otherwise. Touching the skin, one becomes aware of its temperature and texture. The rising and falling of the chest can be felt, as can the patient's breath on one's face. It becomes easy to notice certain details of the skin, its colour, the presence of pigmentation, scars and moles. Pressing down the diaphragm of the stethoscope also creates a sense of the skin's resistance, indicating its age and condition, the presence of muscle, bone and fat.

Just as the physics of the stethoscope suggest that the vibrations of the chest wall are conducted through tubes directly to the ears of the physician,

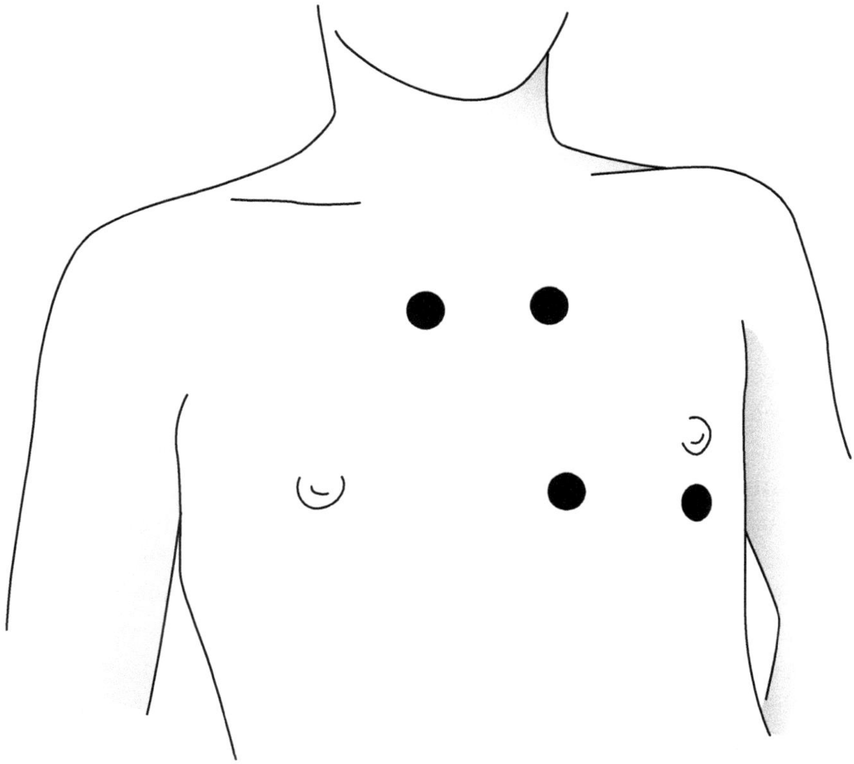

Figure 5 *Key listening points for cardiac auscultation. (Image reproduced with permission of the Queen's University Belfast Clinical Skills Education Centre).*

the sensation for the auscultator is one of a sudden rush of body sounds up the tubes, suffusing the ears. Instead of the doctor penetrating the patient's body with a kind of auditory gaze the sensation is more one of the patient's body penetrating that of the listener. Yost writes that sounds presented over earphones are generally perceived by experimental subjects as being 'inside the head' rather than 'out in space' where actual sound sources usually appear (1994:178). The same is true for the sound conveyed to the earpieces of the stethoscope. Making sense of the cacophony is almost impossible at first. There is only the feeling of something like a sonic draught reaching the head and one becomes overwhelmed, or, as Ellman writes, 'stuffed with sound' (1993:101). This is not to say that the other senses are negated or somehow deleted from experience, but the sense of hearing is given a definite immediacy and priority in the sensory present.

In the earlier lessons of the rotation, few of us could make any sense of what we perceived to be the meaningless 'noise' that invaded our ears. Shaking our heads we apologized to Dr Coltart, saying things like 'I'm sorry, I can't hear anything. I honestly can't hear anything.' As Tom explained:

> When you first come in you don't know what you're listening for. You're just listening. You've got your ears open and everything's coming in and you're like 'Arrrgh!' The first time I came in I didn't know anything. I didn't know what were the heart sounds, I was just listening and thinking 'Oh my God.'

Mary agreed: 'You try to convince yourself that you're hearing something but actually you have no idea.' Like Tom and Mary, many students initially despaired of their inability to control the stethoscope and the sounds produced with it.

Focusing

Dr Coltart encouraged his students to focus and 'listen into' the sounds the stethoscope produced. The type of listening shifted from being directly 'causal' towards what Chion, citing Schaeffer, refers to as 'reduced listening' (Schaeffer 1966:270, cited Chion 1994:29). The emphasis was more 'on the traits of the sound itself, independent of its cause and of its meaning' (ibid.). Many students shut their eyes, screwing them up tight as if attempting forcibly to channel or divert their attention away from their eyes and into their ears. They seemed to be trying to create a sealed perceptual space in which auditory information could be purified and optimized by shutting out potential sensory distractions. Harjit was an eye-closer. 'If you close your eyes you can hear better. You have to suspend all your other senses and put all your energy into your ears,' she said, later referring to this state as 'murmur mode'. Other students kept their eyes open to listen, but stared blankly ahead or into the middle distance as they did so. 'Your eyes may be open but you lose your vision. You stare into space but you don't see anything because your concentration is in your ears,' said Dave. Here the gaze is disengaged. It has been vacated or shut off in order to allow sounds to become the focus of attention. Auscultation, then, requires an unusual acoustic effort, a special kind of concentration, 'a will', as Dave put it, 'to think yourself into your ears'.

In much the same way that experienced concertgoers might close their eyes and let their heads drop back, abandoning themselves to the music, the students' efforts to listen also constituted a kind of performance of listening. This was perhaps helpful in convincing themselves that they were listening as attentively as possible, but it also served to demonstrate to their teacher that they were trying hard and that even if they were not actually able to detect anything meaningful, at least their self-application was good and they were making an effort. Students were later advised that a clear demonstration of listening communicates to the patient that conversation should be suspended and it is time for the doctor to concentrate. This performance of listening therefore served as a technique for both shutting out extraneous sound and distracting presences, and, if necessary, shutting up the patient.

After finding their auditory focus, Dr Coltart told the students to listen for what he called the 'landmark' sounds, the 'lub' and 'dub' that compose the heartbeat. He suggested that if these were soft, then we should nod our heads with each beat, or tap out the rhythm with one foot, thus marking and reinforcing the sounds with bodily movements, lending them a kind of kinaesthetic amplification. He also instructed us to listen while feeling the patient's pulse, not only to anchor the sounds of the heart in tactile sensation but also to check for delays between the heartbeat and the rise of the pulse as these could be of clinical significance. This could involve a kind of sensory cross-referencing, whereby tactile information is used to reinforce that in the auditory mode. After a few lessons most of us were able to recognize the 'lub' and 'dub' with some degree of certainty, although we periodically encountered patients whose heart sounds were indiscernible to us.

Next Dr Coltart asked us to listen for heart murmurs and other abnormal heart sounds. He used both a temporal and a visual-spatial framework in order to describe the auditory focus that is necessary. To start with, he suggested that we try devoting units of time to the elements of what we were hearing:

> There's no way that you can hear all of the information that's there in one go. You've got to have points that you're listening for and that you can work from. You've got to listen for five seconds to everything, then for five seconds you've got to find the heart sounds, then you've got to listen for five seconds for any murmurs before or after those sounds.

He also suggested that we mark the first and second heart sounds using imaginary lines, and then, if additional sounds could be detected, draw or shade in the spaces on either side of the first or second heart sounds in which they occurred (see Figure 6). He depicted murmurs in this way on notepads and blackboards. This diagrammatic formulation of sounds was helpful to students who were not accustomed to working in sound alone and found it easier to visualize them. Dr Coltart claimed, however, that as one becomes familiarized with heart sounds and more confident at recognizing the different kinds of murmurs, one ceases to rely on mental images. Instead there is an automatic auditory recognition.

Evidence from psychoacoustics suggests that people are able to separate specific 'acoustic objects' from their background, isolating particular elements

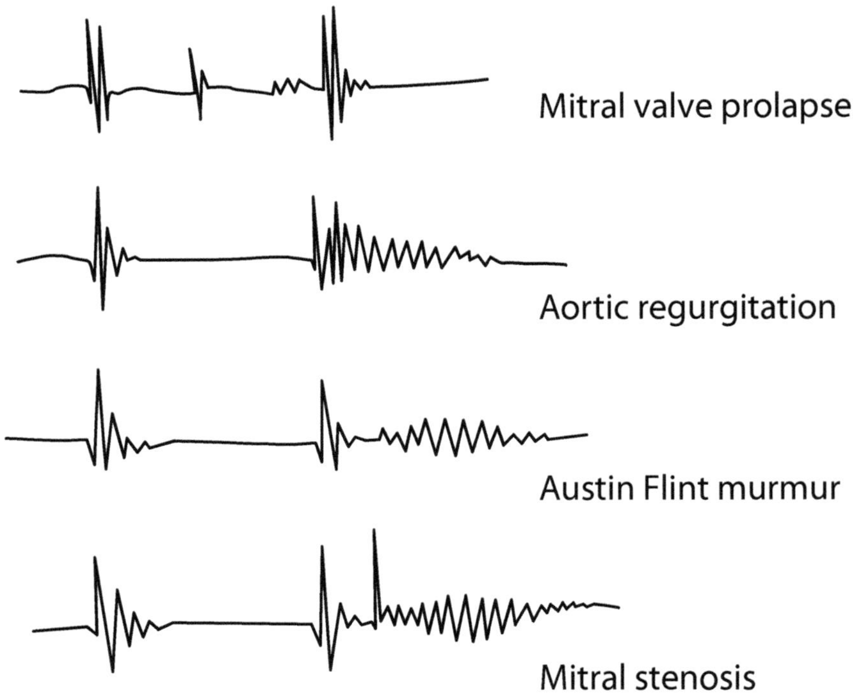

Figure 6 *Heart murmur sketches.*

for focused attention. Indeed, the ear works by attending to parts of complex sounds, rather than all aspects at once. As Moore explains:

> It seems that we are not generally capable of attending to every aspect of the auditory input...rather, certain points are selected for conscious analysis... it appears that the complex sound signal is analysed into streams, and we attend primarily to one stream at a time. This attended stream then stands out perceptually, while the rest of the sound is less prominent (2003:294–5).

It may be that Dr Coltart's system for spatially and temporally demarcating the different parts of a sound facilitates this process of 'streaming'. Moore also identifies distinct 'analytic' or 'synthetic' modes of hearing. The 'analytic' mode allows the listener to attend to individual components of a sound, thus effectively muting other parts, while the 'synthetic' mode fuses elements into a single percept (ibid.:282). Warren suggests that an element of training may be necessary in order for listeners to shift effectively between the 'analytic' and 'synthetic' modes (1982:63). Following an experiment in which a series of tones were played to doctors through a stethoscope, Welsby, Parry, and Smith (2003) noted that practised auscultators were effective at filtering out extraneous or misleading sounds. This suggests that they had become adept at shifting between the analytic and synthetic modes of hearing.

Listening alone together

Daniel Shindler (2004) remarks upon students' 'enthusiasm for the stethoscope' when introduced to auscultation. Indeed, my fellow students were surprisingly keen to practise listening to murmurs. At Dr Coltart's suggestion they visited the cardiothoracic wards after class, asking nurses on duty if there were any murmur patients to whom they might listen. They returned repeatedly to see patients whose murmurs were challenging. The consequences of this repeated listening for the patients is a subject I discuss in the following chapter. But despite their general enthusiasm, students nevertheless experienced difficulties with learning to listen.

In many learning contexts, for instance those described by Marchand (2010b) and Makovicky (2010), the physical substance of materials with which teachers and pupils work (wood and thread respectively) is shown to be integral to the teaching process. Participants in the teaching interactions appear to have a strong visual, tactile, and even olfactory engagement with the materials. At the same time, the student's work with and upon that material indicates how well particular actions and techniques are being performed, and hence how well the student is progressing. Wood and thread bear the physical traces of the practitioner's skills (or lack of them), and hence can easily be made the subject of comparison and discussion. The medical students, on the other hand, found it difficult to establish common points of reference for the sounds they were hearing and it was difficult to gauge or have confidence in their own progress as listeners.

Auscultation is considered a solitary, isolating perceptual experience. This is partly because stethoscopic listening, like the iPod listening described by, for instance, Bull (2000), is privatized. The sounds of the body are narrowcast – channelled through earpieces – not broadcast into public space. The students could never be sure that they were hearing the sound Dr. Coltart wanted them to be hearing or whether they were making some mistake in their placement of the stethoscope. Technologies have been developed to get around this problem. Teaching stethoscopes with as many as ten pairs of earpieces leading off a single central diaphragm (ensuring that everyone is listening to the same sound) are available, and recently, digital stethoscopes have been produced that allow heart sounds to be amplified, recorded, and played back. However, while they are available to purchase, I did not see either of these devices in use at St. Thomas'. At the time of writing, the smartphone application iStethoscope Pro became available. This software allows heart sounds to be recorded and played back into shared auditory space via the phone's speakers.

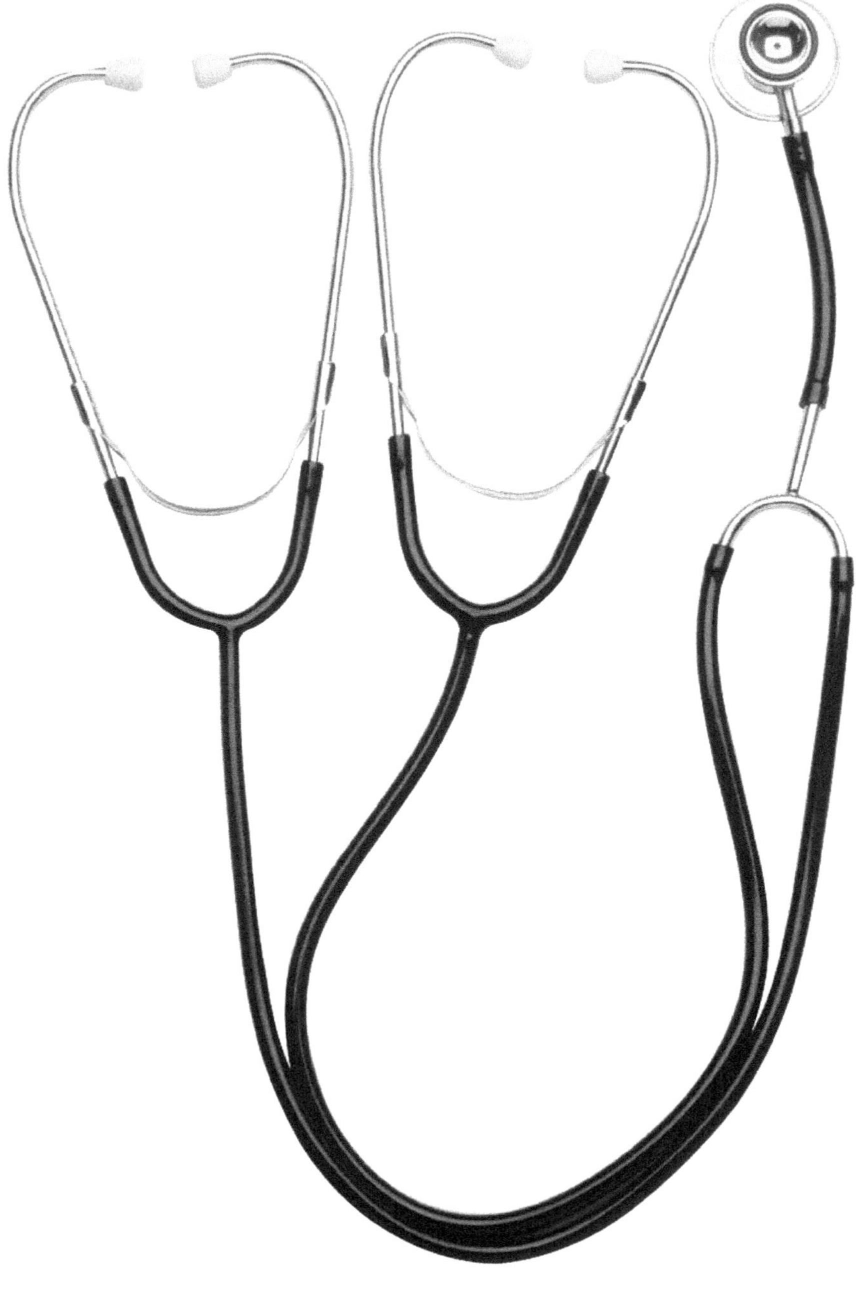

Figure 7 *A teaching stethoscope. Reproduced with permission of St John Ambulance Supplies.*

Filters can be applied to make the desired frequencies of the heart sound clearer and to minimize background noise. A key benefit of this application is its capacity to make heart sounds easy to share between listeners. This technology only emerged after my time at St Thomas', however, so I never saw it used there. Auscultation was always a solitary endeavour, the doctor or student listening to sounds that he or she alone could hear. The listener was isolated in a particular perceptual moment.

One way in which Dr Coltart, and teaching doctors more generally, sought to get around the problem of the subjective isolation of listening was to provide students with CD recordings of various murmurs. Professionally produced by a major stethoscope manufacturer, this set of recordings included voice-overs naming each individual heart sound and describing its particular sonic characteristics. Students found the CD helpful. It enabled them to listen collectively during classes, boosting confidence that they were hearing what they were meant to hear and not sounds produced by their own mishandling or misplacement of the stethoscope. Dr Coltart also wanted students to be capable of instantly recognizing some of the most common heart murmurs, 'as one knows a dog's bark'. The ejection systolic murmur of aortic stenosis, for example, occurs when the aortic valve becomes stiffened and no longer opens fully enough to allow easy blood flow. As a consequence, the blood is forced through the narrowed valve, resulting in a distinctive, harsh, sometimes squeaky murmur. The CD familiarized students with such archetypal examples, and with other common heart sounds. They were then able to compare murmurs heard on the wards with these memorized sounds. Whenever they detected subtle or more unusual sounds, they were also able to refer to the recorded examples as a kind of sonic template.

CD recordings detach heart murmurs from patients, effectively turning the sounds into portable sonic objects. Practice listening was therefore no longer restricted to the hospital, freeing students to learn the sounds in their own bedrooms or while travelling to and from class. This also released them from the pressure they felt when listening in Dr Coltart's presence. Some listened to the CD while reading, which they claimed allowed the murmurs gradually to seep into the memory rather than being forcibly memorized. A few students visited websites where they could listen to heart murmur recordings and view phonocardiograms (digitally produced diagrams of heart sounds). These effectively served the same purpose as the classroom sketches drawn by Dr Coltart, though they tended to be more detailed, colourful, and aesthetically pleasing for the students (Figure 8).

Though considered to be helpful, the recorded sounds are much 'bigger' and 'cleaner' than those received through a stethoscope. In live listening sounds can be muddled and obscured by subcutaneous fat, vascular noise and

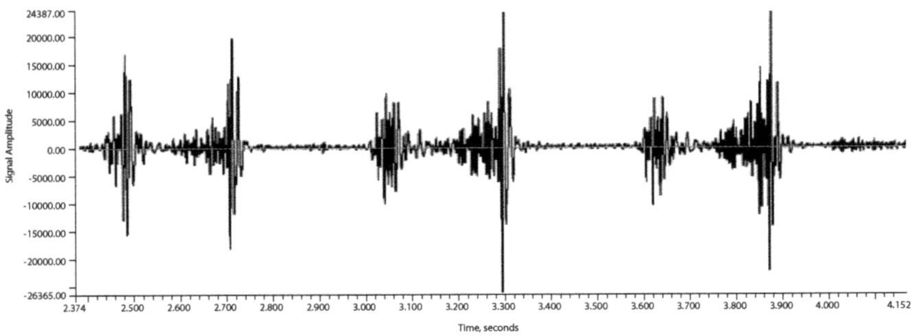

Figure 8 *A phonocardiogram of the murmur of mitral regurgitation. (Image reproduced with permission of Bsignetics).*

breath sounds from inside the body. Recordings and sound files generally lack the background noises of the wider ward/patient context as well as the realism of the stethoscope-user interface. After several days of listening, students could reliably complete the 'heart sound quiz' at the end of the CD, but finding and recognizing the same murmurs through a stethoscope when faced with a live patient proved more challenging and required many weeks of practice. Even by the end of the rotation no student was consistently successful in this task.

Speaking sound

The teaching of auscultation also presents a linguistic problem, or a problem of vocabulary. While the previously mentioned ethnographies by Feld, Gell, and Weiner point to the highly sophisticated acoustic vocabularies exhibited by members of the Papuan societies they study, sonic terminology is generally held to be comparatively under-developed in Western societies. It is not simply that there is a 'Spartan economy of words' for engaging with auditory phenomena, but that, as Murch argues, Western cultures have never developed the concepts or language to describe or cope with sound (Marchand 2010a:7; Murch 1994:xvi–xvii).

While standing at the bedside of patients, Dr Coltart often tried to produce evocative descriptions of particular heart sounds for his students, saying things like: 'It's that long, low, rumbling sound I want you to be getting,' or 'Can you hear that harsh, rasping, almost squeaking sound?' While terms like 'lub dub,' and even 'murmur,' are clearly onomatopoeic, Dr Coltart also resorted to more conspicuous forms of mimicry. 'It's the "ush, ush, ush" I want you to listen to,' he might say, or the 'lup dup shh, lub dup shh.' On several occasions Dr Coltart acted out the murmur of aortic stenosis by saying 'eek, eek, eek,' accenting the noise with an upward gesture of his fist to indicate the effort required to pump blood through the narrowed valve.

In a similar way, Birdsall (2009) describes how people she interviewed about their sound memories of the Nazi period frequently resorted to making noises and gestures in order to articulate auditory experiences they were not able to express in words. The medical students often used onomatopoeia in describing what they heard to one another. The performance of sounds and use of nonsense words and syllables often had a comic effect, partly because of their perceived contrast with the serious manner and formal terminology that supposedly characterized clinical discussions. However, these vocalizations were another attempt to break down the subjective isolation of listening and make the stethoscopic auditory experience a shared and communal one through public language and gesture.

One of the linguistic devices used by Laennec to evoke the sounds that he heard in his patients and which he wanted other doctors to recognize was simile. As indicated in Chapter 3, he described one particular lung sound as 'a tinkling similar to that of a small bell just ceasing to ring, or of a fly buzzing in a china vase' (1846:320). Elsewhere he described how the thickening of the bronchial tubes caused by pneumonia yielded a sound that sometimes resembled snoring, the cooing of a wood pigeon, or the rubbing of a bass string (Marks 1972:71–2). Such acoustic analogies have largely disappeared from modern medical descriptions of heart sounds, but Dr Coltart nevertheless made reference to, for example, a 'seagull murmur' and 'a gallop rhythm'. He suggested that the gallop rhythm, which is produced when a third heart sound is audible in addition to the expected two, should have the same cadence as the word 'Kentucky', the first heart sound forming the 'Ken', the second heart sound the 'tuc', and the third sound the 'ky'. The rhythm produced when a fourth heart sound is present was likened to the word 'Tennessee'. While a third heart sound comes after the two expected ones, the fourth heart sound precedes them. Interestingly, a third heart sound is not required for a fourth to be present, so in the three syllables of 'Tennessee' the fourth heart sound makes the 'Tenn', the first the 'ess', and the second the 'ee'. By invoking more familiar acoustic patterns, these metaphors make otherwise inchoate sounds more immediately comprehensible (Fernandez 1974:120).

Doctors at St Thomas' would define heart murmurs using a set of four parameters. They might refer, for instance, to 'a soft, grade II ejection-systolic murmur at the left sternal edge'. The murmur is thereby classified in terms of its tone, volume (on a scale of I to VI), place in the cardiac cycle and location on the chest. This method greatly reduces the scope for possible confusion arising from attempts to evoke the actual sound of the murmur. It should be pointed out, however, that the ability to frame sounds through a set of reference-points has not entirely resolved the problem of establishing consensus on what has been heard. Murmurs can be very subtle. Also, like other kinds of diagnostic work, auscultation is interpretative or hermeneutic. Despite efforts to 'fix' murmurs objectively through careful description, it is still common for doctors to disagree on the nature of what can be heard. In an excerpt on 'the heart sounds', *The Oxford Handbook of Clinical Medicine* states that '[t]he first and second sounds are usually clear'; however '[c]onfident pronouncements about the other sounds and soft murmurs may be difficult. Even senior colleagues disagree with one another about the more difficult murmurs.' (Longmore, Wilkinson and Torok 2001:80). In auscultation, sounds still cannot be reliably or unproblematically codified.

Sinclair observes that heart murmurs 'are notoriously hard for novices to identify' (1997:202). But despite the complexities involved in learning to listen, the students gradually increased their proficiency at detecting and interpreting heart sounds. They began to acquire the knowledge of sounds and the specialized auditory skills which auscultation demands. This came with applying the pedagogic techniques invented by doctors, but above all, with practice. Progression was not uniform. As Downey points out, expertise arises in diverse fashion and unevenly (2010). But as one student, Alistair, put it, 'When we started we could hear a sound and that was about it. Then we could hear the two heartbeats and a load of muffle. Now we can listen to that muffle and usually understand what it means.'

Harder hearing

A few months into fieldwork my right ear became itchy and painful, and my hearing a trifle impaired. It seemed likely that I had caught something from a stethoscope. The earpieces are known to be a site at which pathogens accumulate, and people who share stethoscopes often develop ear infections. I had used a spare ward stethoscope on a number of occasions and so now was obliged to return to the hospital as an outpatient.

When I walked into the waiting room of the ENT (Ear, Nose and Throat) Department, I was surprised to see one of the students I had met on the chest rotation. Rhydd was equally surprised to see me. He explained that his ears felt continually blocked and he was finding it increasingly difficult to hear, so he had come to have them syringed. I explained my own reason for attending the clinic, and he told me all about the doctor I would be seeing. It turned out that he had been one of Rhydd's teachers. While we were talking together, Rhydd nodded and smiled at a girl walking past.

> 'Who's that?' I asked.
>
> 'Her name is Nirit. She's a third-year medic as well. She's going into the audiology clinic which is not surprising – she's deaf.'

This was interesting, and I wondered how she coped with the auditory practices that I understood to be so important to medicine. I asked Rhydd if he could arrange a meeting.

Nirit and I met a few days later in the café at St Thomas'. In speaking to her, I was in no way aware of her deafness and did not have to make any concessions in terms of altering my speech. She described herself as 'hearing-impaired' and explained that few people are totally deaf. She considers herself representative of that grey zone within the population who live between deafness and a totally hearing world. Nirit's hearing impediment is congenital. She has 70 per cent hearing loss in each ear, but explained: 'It isn't that I don't hear. I have found strategies to hear in spite of my impediment.' She wears hearing aids and lip-reads. Nirit went on to describe how she made the choice to live as a hearing person in a hearing world. This decision met with disapproval from some members of a group with which she worked. They expected her to assume a 'Deaf' identity and maintain solidarity with other Deaf people by refusing to adapt to the hearing world. Sacks (1989) observes the strength of this ideology among some deaf people in his book *Seeing Voices*.

Nirit acknowledged that there are certain features of medical practice that make the path difficult for the hearing-impaired. Medics spend considerable time attending to weak or elderly people who often speak in a soft, unclear manner. Nirit is also aware that she is easily thrown by accents and unusual words, and hospital background noise further impedes concentrated listening. In the operating theatre, much of the face, including the mouth, is covered, thereby concealing lips, facial expression and normal self-evidence of the speaker, making comprehension especially challenging. Though strategies may be employed (in the operating theatre, for example, surgeons can be asked to wear small radio microphones which relay their voices to a hearing aid), the numerous existing hurdles suggest that medicine is likely to remain a testing career for the hard-of-hearing. There is perhaps an inherent 'audism', which Sterne describes as 'an ethnocentrism of those who hear', within medical culture (2003a:28).

For Nirit, four areas of medicine stood out as highly 'auditory' in nature or rather as being specializations in which listening is especially important. These are general practice, paediatrics, respiratory medicine, and cardiology. Nirit's hearing impairment made her reluctant to go into any of these areas, and cardiology in particular. She would find it hard to cope with the responsibility were she were unable to detect a sound that was an important diagnostic clue and jeopardize a patient's health as a consequence. 'I don't want to spend all my life wondering if a patient's well-being has been compromised by my hearing,' she said.

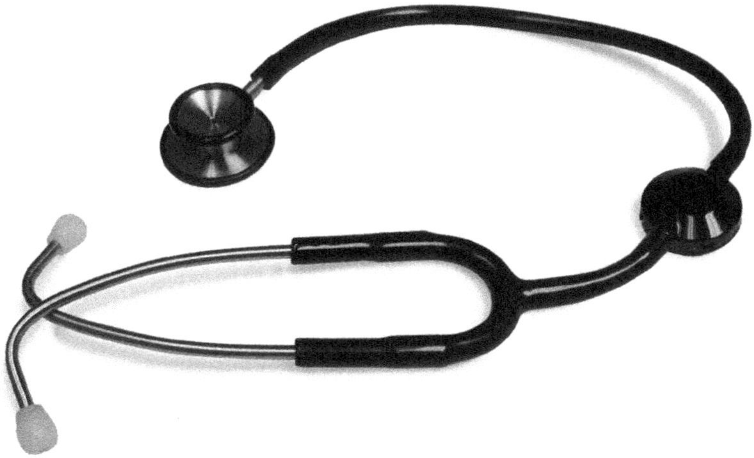

Figure 9 *An amplified stethoscope. Reproduced with permission of Harris Communications, Inc.: http://www.harriscomm.com.*

The 'chest rotation' included instruction in the rudiments of two of the most acoustically demanding specialisms, namely respiratory medicine and cardiology. A great deal of auscultation practice was demanded in these elements of the training, and the technique presented obvious challenges to Nirit. She acquired an amplified stethoscope (see Figure 9) which was manufactured in such a way that the main tube extending from the diaphragm plugs into a small amplifier that, in turn, is connected to the earpieces. The sound picked up by the diaphragm travels up the tube, is amplified half way and continues in normal fashion to the earpieces. In addition to making the sounds from patients louder, the device can also be tuned to amplify high or low frequencies.

Nirit had been anxious about auscultation. She pointed out that she was used to listening because the fact that her *hearing* is impaired makes *listening* all the more important. She must actively seek out the sounds most people hear easily and take for granted. In everyday life, Nirit used lip-reading and other cues to fill in for missing sounds. In auscultation, however, supporting information was not immediately available, leaving her sense of hearing uncomfortably exposed. She explained that her amplified stethoscope also worried her because she did not know whether it was distorting sounds. She thought she might be hearing things that were not there. This feeling is reported by almost all students who learn auscultation, but Nirit believed the problem to be more acute in her case, undermining her confidence in judging what she heard.

One teaching doctor offered Nirit extra one-to-one supervision in auscultation. He took her around the wards to practise listening on patients with exemplary heart murmurs and gave her more time to listen than she received during normal classes. Nirit found the technique of tapping or acting out elements of the sounds with gestures particularly helpful. She believed that doing this, even if only in her head, was a good way of confirming to herself the acoustic dynamics of the sounds she was detecting. She also appreciated the care taken by the teaching doctor to describe and mimic sounds accurately. She felt that this process of verbalization provided a way of moving the sounds out of her perceptual uncertainty into a space in which their features and characteristics could be shared and thereby verified.

By taking turns at listening and afterwards comparing thoughts, the teaching doctor and Nirit were together able to analyse and monitor her hearing. The teaching doctor directed Nirit's attention to areas of relative perceptual strength and weakness. He advised her to pay particular attention to certain parts of sounds and to trust her judgement on others. Gradually, Nirit's ear for heart murmurs became more reliable. The perceptual isolation she experienced, 'amplified' by the amplified stethoscope, was slowly dispelled, giving way to relative confidence. Her faith in both the technology and her own sense of hearing grew. By the end of the chest rotation, Nirit recognized that although some fellow students were better skilled, some were less competent than her. This was in fact the case for every rotation, not just those that drew heavily on auditory skills.

To use her amplified stethoscope, Nirit had first to remove her hearing aids and insert the earpieces of the instrument, listen, and then take them out and reinsert her hearing aids. While this would be fine for her medical exams, she felt that in a normal medical setting the same procedure might undermine patients' confidence in her diagnostic abilities. A report entitled *Enabling Disabled Doctors* suggests that doctors with visible disabilities of all kinds occasionally encounter assumptions of incompetence made by patients (Morgan and Chambers 2004). Nirit was concerned that patients might not realise that, in fact, her hearing is sufficient for carrying out her duties. While becoming confident with her use of the stethoscope, she nevertheless recognized that she would need to be creative in managing patient reactions to her methods and securing their trust.

The amplified stethoscope allows Nirit to use auscultation in the same way as other medical students, but the technique continues to hold greater challenges for her than for most of her peers. Nirit's example demonstrates that bodies, and the perceptual capacities they support, are not uniform or homogeneous, but are sites for the production of difference. Nirit's hearing problems do not prevent her from participating in what might be described as the 'common schemes of perception' that characterize a medical habitus (Bourdieu 1980:60). She can assemble the same 'body techniques', the same 'body hexis', as other students and doctors. But plainly, thinking in these terms could lead us to dismiss what is important and interesting in Nirit's example, namely that certain tasks are more problematic and fraught with doubt and uncertainty for her than for other students. Her sense of hearing requires that she be unusually careful, conscientious, inventive and resourceful in her approach to her medical training.

'A difficult skill to acquire'

On one hand, this chapter shows that doctors are inventive, resourceful and ultimately quite successful at imparting the auditory knowledge which stethoscopic listening demands. They have developed a combination of techniques that productively direct the novice's auditory attention, memory and recognition, and by practising in the learning environment of a hospital ward the listening skills of most medical students progress and will continue to develop. On the other hand, my research also reinforces the point that auscultation is 'a difficult skill to acquire' (Roy 2009:4). The amount of practice and repetition required makes the skill costly in terms of both time and energy for teachers and students alike. The inherent subjectivity of auditory experience and judgement, as well as the difficulty of fluent and confident communication about sounds has made auscultation problematic for doctors since its inception. The challenges and constraints of listening as a way of knowing are made apparent in its transmission. Indeed, those challenges and constraints become particularly pronounced and are repeatedly confronted, realized and enacted in auscultation classes.

As discussed in more detail in Chapter 8, on a number of occasions I heard senior doctors remark that the stethoscope was 'a dying technology' and auscultation 'a dying art'. They pointed to the increasing use of cardiac ultrasound or echocardiography in heart examinations and consequent diagnoses of heart disease. A number of written sources also make reference to the 'death of the stethoscope', again pointing to the impact of new technologies on diagnostic practice (e.g. Babu 1999; Kirsch 1998). While techniques such as echocardiography will present their own sets of problems and complexities as ways of knowing, doctors may ultimately consider these to be more acceptable or manageable than those involved in stethoscopic listening. It is possible that doctors will begin to resist using and teaching auscultation in clinical practice as alternative, less demanding and training-intensive diagnostic technologies emerge.

Downey writes that 'our species' remarkable ability to learn derives not merely from our intelligence as learners, but also from our skill as teachers' (2010:28). This remark is optimistic, even congratulatory. Such a tone is almost irresistible when contemplating the wide and varied range of skills humans are able to acquire and pass on to others. The doctors with whom I worked did indeed demonstrate impressive practical intelligence in enacting pedagogic strategies for the teaching of stethoscopic listening. The doctor who took responsibility for coaching Nirit also showed admirable personal dedication and patience in tailoring his instruction to her particular sensory needs and abilities. It is important to point out that doctors also continue to seek solutions to the difficulties of teaching and learning, for instance by designing technological aids and incorporating them into training. It may be that the iStethoscope application, for example, will be highly successful in this regard, and that rather than signalling the end of stethoscopic listening it will give the technique new life and expand its possibilities. The potential for smart phones to allow the display of sound waveforms and to amplify body sounds may also increase students' speed and efficiency in learning auscultation (though it is possible, too, that these capacities of the technology may render fine listening skills unnecessary). At the time of my research, however, the medical profession had been unable decisively to overcome the challenges of auscultation and the difficulties presented by the transmission of this kind of auditory knowledge. It may be that, in clinical settings like the Cardiothoracic Unit at St Thomas', the complexities of teaching and learning cardiac auscultation ultimately make the continued use of the technique difficult to justify, meaning that its importance will gradually diminish and it will ultimately disappear from the daily skill set of doctors and students.

CHAPTER 6

'Beautiful Murmurs'

Stethoscopic Listening and Acoustic Objectification

In clinics that focused on the chest examination and the use of auscultation, heart murmurs were of particular interest. In the sessions in which I took part, Dr Coltart would try to select patients with distinctive murmurs for his students to listen to. He emphasized to students the importance of 'listening again', of going back to listen to patients with exemplary murmurs several times to be sure that the sounds became familiar and that they would recognize them in future. Occasionally, doctors identified what they described as a 'classic' or 'beautiful' murmur, typical of a particular type of heart disease. Patients with such murmurs could be very useful in the teaching of auscultation and doctors would ask them if they would be happy to participate in classes. As I explain below, there is a culture within the hospital of patients being used in teaching and few patients ever refused this request, meaning that several groups of students might listen to a patient's heart in a single day. This repeated auscultation often had an effect on patients. They felt that doctors and students tended to look, or in this case listen, past them as persons, focusing instead on their diagnostic signs. Their bodies, and the murmurs within their bodies, underwent a process of objectification through auscultation.

The term 'objectification' has two separate but related meanings. The first refers to a capacity to make external and concrete, and hence situate as perceptually 'objective'. The second relates to the tendency to regard a being as an 'object', hence treating it impersonally and abstractly and rendering it liable to manipulation or control. Visual perception has been linked to objectification in both these senses. For instance, it has been argued that vision by necessity involves the creation of perceptual distance, so externalizing that which is perceived and making it objective (Carpenter 1976, Classen 1998). At the same time, vision and acts of gazing have become integral to theories of the objectification of persons. Thus, the male gaze has become associated with the objectification of the female body and its reinvention as a sexualized being-for-men rather than a being-for-itself (Berger 1972, Mulvey 1975, Jordanova 1989, Grosz 1992).

The link between sight and 'objectification' in both related senses of the term has grown strong, so that visual perceptual practices have tended to be regarded as intrinsically objectifying. Audition and listening, on the other hand, have often been imagined to create an intimate and participatory form of sensory engagement that does not produce objectification (Stoller 1989, Gell 1995). This chapter explores how some patients become acutely conscious of the way in which clinical auscultation reifies their heart sounds, constructing murmurs as discrete acoustic objects inside their bodies. If listening is frequently repeated, patients feel objectified as clinical curiosities. In addition to engaging with patient experiences, the chapter also briefly considers a separate but related context in which auscultation is involved in the sexual objectification of the female body. It is argued that the notion that objectification may be brought about through an acoustic practice invites a reappraisal of the perceptual possibilities of audition.

The chapter develops a theme which runs throughout this book, namely that sound and ways of listening are constitutive of the doctor-patient relationship in complex and often unexpected ways. It shows how patients' involvement in teaching sessions and subsequent repeated auscultation is at best semi-voluntary, framing the doctor-patient interaction as an obligation resulting from patients' participation in a nationalized healthcare system. The chapter also reveals how repeated auscultation can entail a deaf ear being turned to all but the patient's diagnostic signs, situating the doctor-patient relationship simply as an association between the doctor and a particular pathology or diseased part of the patient's body. Finally, it examines circumstances in which auscultation allows the doctor-patient relationship to become loaded with sexual frisson.

The sight/hearing dichotomy

In *The Audible Past*, Sterne identifies what he calls an 'audiovisual litany', a set of assertions which he observes are repeatedly made about the difference between hearing and vision (2003a:15). The following are among the contrasts listed by Sterne, although his litany is more extensive:

> Hearing immerses its subject, vision offers a perspective.
> Hearing places us inside an event, seeing gives us a perspective on the event.
> Hearing tends towards subjectivity, vision towards objectivity.
> Hearing is about affect, vision is about intellect.

For Sterne, these differences 'are often considered as biological, psychological, and physical facts' (ibid.). The litany, he suggests, is adopted by numerous authors un-reflexively, without consideration of the historical and 'ideological baggage' it carries with it (ibid.:16). Referring to this set of sensory contrasts as a 'litany' is appropriate, Sterne argues, because it in fact has its origins in Christian and to some extent pre-Christian thought. He points to a 'longstanding spirit/letter distinction', in which the spirit is living and life giving, leading to salvation, and the letter is dead and inert, leading to damnation (ibid.). Spirit and letter each have what Sterne calls 'sensory analogues', so that hearing leads a soul to spirit, while sight leads a soul to letter (ibid.). He suggests that the essential notion that 'the sonic dimension of experience is closest to divinity' while vision 'suggests distance and disengagement' percolates influential work on the senses, his case in point being Ong's (1982) *Orality and Literacy* (ibid.:17).

In a similar way, Leach observes that 'the idea that vision is objectifying and distancing, whereas sound is subjective, immediate and experiential, is quite familiar to Western sensibility' (2003:203). He considers this notion to have influenced writing and thought on the senses within anthropology and uses the work of Gell (1995) and Stoller (1989) to illustrate this point. For both these ethnographers, distance separates the perceiving subject from the perceived object in the act of looking, producing discrete objects. Hearing, on the other hand, creates an 'intimate, concrete and tactile' sensory engagement (Gell 1995:235). Leach considers that both Gell and Stoller produce insightful analyses of their respective ethnographic contexts. However, he is also conscious that they have imposed 'a direct contrast in the functioning of alternative sensory modalities' upon their non-Western ethnography 'as though it was simply a given' (2003:203).

The pre-supposition of a link between sight and objectivity has led to vision being regarded as in itself responsible for the creation and reproduction of particular cultural practices. For instance, vision is held to have been the key to the development of Western science because, as Carpenter puts it, 'sight has a natural bias toward detachment, creating the detached observer' (1976:40). For Classen, sight 'carries with it a powerful aura of rationality and objectivity' which encourages 'the exercise of reason' (Classen 1998:1). The objectifying gaze is understood to provide the perceptual basis of Western rationalism.

Being so closely associated with the Western 'world-view', the sense of sight has also been identified as the root of what are perceived to be negative traits endemic in Western hegemony (Ong 1969). Stoller (1997), for instance, argues that Western visualism has led to a tendency towards detachment and analysis that precludes an appreciation of more participatory and sensorially immediate types of engagement with the world as practised and experienced by other cultures. Fabian (1983) points out that the visual basis of Western perceptual schemes has created limited and reductive ways of organizing and representing social life. Theorists have tended, then, to reify the sense of sight itself, attributing to it an independent agency and endowing it with a (largely negative) 'personality' of its own: one which, through its perceived propensity to objectify, has fostered distinct and what many consider to be flawed cultural forms.

A different point of view is provided by Bubandt, who warns that 'one should not exaggerate the "inherent" hegemonic potential of any particular sense' (1998:66). He argues that the hegemony of vision has never been monolithic or complete in the West, and has, in any case, created possibilities for 'counter-visions' that may potentially challenge an established visual order (ibid.:68). Bubandt observes that a consideration of the consequences of a perceived Western 'visualism' has also led to a search for other, more benign perceptual groundings for knowledge and power (ibid.:49). However, in relation to his own area of interest – the anthropology of smell and olfactory knowledge – he points out that 'attempts to topple the taken-for-granted primacy of vision by descriptions of "exotic" uses of smell' have 'tended to present us with a radical alterity free from the "vices of vision" rather than with a detailed political ontology of a culturally specific mode of olfaction' (ibid.). Bubandt's suggestion is that studies of olfactory perception have tended to be carried out with the aim of destabilizing a demonized visual hegemony. Such studies, however, do not give careful consideration to the actual character and implications of the olfactory perceptual strategies and systems they claim to explore. Sight is, as it were, 'put in the black hat' in order to set up a critical trajectory for rather superficial analyses of olfactory practices.

Theorists writing on auditory perceptual practices have also claimed to define benign alternatives to Western visualism. Gell points towards hearing as a sense of emotional and evocative immediacy creating 'cultures of sympathy' (1995:235). Again, the qualities of hearing as identified by Sterne in the audiovisual litany are strongly in evidence here. More esoteric thinkers have suggested that, by using audition over sight, people become more spiritual, better connected to subtle but fundamental vibratory presences in the world. In his book *The World is Sound*, Berendt describes the eyes as 'aggressive, dominating, rational, surface-oriented, analyzing things' whereas the ears are 'female, receptive, careful, intuitive, spiritual, depth-oriented, perceiving the whole as one' (1983:5). Berendt suggests that wisdom and harmony might be produced through the widespread adoption of an auditory orientation towards the world. This would be preferable, in his view, to what he sees as the relentless recourse to aggressive forms of analytical abstraction that have been the consequence of visual culture.

The example of auscultation indicates that hearing does not necessarily or logically create a type of intimate, inclusive and participatory perceptual experience. Neither is it inherently productive of cultural forms that are free from what might be described as the objectifying 'vices of vision'. This chapter, and indeed the book as a whole, seeks to challenge any such assumptions about the nature of auditory perception, and avoids making an appeal to any apparently 'natural' and trans-historical qualities of the sense of hearing. It regards auscultation as itself encultured, the product of a particular field of socio-historical currents within Western medicine. It positions the technique as one in which the sense of hearing is channelled in the interests of science, reason and rationality, clear imperatives of the medical culture of Western Europe in the nineteenth century.

It is also important to point out that while the term 'objectification' may have negative connotations through its association with power and control, it has also been conceptualized as a constructive and indeed necessary perceptual step in the production of knowledge and in the organization of thought and action. Thus, Lewis (2000) argues that the objectification of the body in Western medicine is fundamental to the identification and ultimately the treatment of disease. Jackson (1994) also points to patients' objectification of their own body parts and processes, which he suggests is an essential step in enabling them to conceptualize the diseases by which they are affected, ultimately allowing them to manage their symptoms. This chapter situates auscultation as involved in productive forms of medical objectification that enable, for instance, heart sounds to be constructed as diagnostic signs. But it also explains that in the context of teaching sessions, repeated auscultation can lead to distinct, negatively experienced forms of objectification through which patients generally understand themselves to have been reduced to clinically interesting acoustic objects.

The position of patients

Patients were alerted to the presence of students, potentially during all stages of their treatment, through the *Guy's and St Thomas' Outpatient Leaflet*. At the time of my fieldwork, the leaflet read:

> Both Guy's and St Thomas' are teaching hospitals, responsible for training a wide range of health professionals. This means that students, supervised by qualified staff, might be involved in your care. It does not affect the quality of your care in any way, but does give valuable training for the students.
>
> Please tell the doctor or nurse in charge if you do not want students to be present. Your wishes will always be respected.

This text underscores how beneficial it is for students to be taught, so to speak 'using' patients.

As indicated earlier in the book, Foucault (1973) describes how in the eighteenth century the hospital as an institution came to comprise both a place of care for the sick poor, and a place in which doctors and students of medicine received practical training. Foucault notes the 'hidden contract' that was formed around the seemingly comfortable fit of this dual purpose (ibid.:83). In return for the care they were to receive in the hospital, patients would be obliged to make themselves available for use in medical training. Foucault questions the morality of this arrangement, and even suggests that positioning patients as teaching material involves the enactment of a subtle violence: 'to show in order to teach, is this not a tacit form of violence...upon a sick body that demands to be comforted, not displayed?' (ibid.:84). He points out that the position of the poor patient as 'an object of clinical observation' in the late eighteenth century was brought about through his charitable status within the hospital. 'Can pain be a spectacle? Not only can it be, but it must be, by virtue of a subtle right that resides in the fact that no one is alone, the poor man less so than others, since he can attain assistance only through the mediation of the rich' (ibid.). The patient is entrapped by 'the tyranny of the gift', effectively coerced into being used in the education of students through his indebtedness to those by whom care is provided (Fox and Swazey 1992:40).

Richardson (1987) describes how in the early nineteenth century, the poor patient would be obliged to come to the hospital (she specifically mentions St Thomas') 'cap in hand, to beg relief from the pain of his affliction; and finding this great institution willing to open its doors, would be expected to be duly grateful' (ibid.:47). A wealthy patient would be unlikely to go to a hospital and was in a position to assess the reputation of various doctors, dismissing or refusing to pay those who did not provide satisfactory treatment. Poor patients, however, constituted a passive clientele, unable to challenge the aims and demands of the doctors who took charge of their cases. They would therefore provide a 'source of clinical material' which was 'also cast in the role of human *teaching* material' (ibid.; original emphasis). Poor patients provided the means through which paying medical students could acquire experience and observe medical techniques.

Medicine has certainly undergone huge changes since the time to which both Foucault and Richardson refer, but it is clear that some fundamental social structures have remained constant. The system for the funding of public hospitals has largely shifted from one based solely on charitable donations and patronage to a more complex model of mainly government provision. In both the St Thomas' of 1828 described by Richardson and the St Thomas' of 2003–4 that I encountered during fieldwork, however, there was the same general assumption that patients could be 'used' in the education of students. As the extracts from the leaflet cited above make clear, it is presumed that patients admitted to St Thomas' will accept, or at least will only in exceptional cases not accept, their role as 'teaching material'.

The vast majority of patients I encountered during fieldwork did indeed agree to be involved in teaching. Some felt that by allowing themselves to be examined as part of classes they were helping to train the next generation of doctors, making a contribution to the care others would receive in years to come. 'They've got to learn some time, haven't they?' was a commonly expressed sentiment. 'I should do my little bit to help them, after all, they're the doctors of the future!' Other patients said that they were glad to be useful. Rather than existing solely as a burden on the hospital, absorbing its resources, they could now do something to help and thus make a small gesture of reciprocation for all the care they had received. Some patients also enjoyed having something to do after spending long periods of time on the ward feeling bored and useless. In an environment where there is often a lot of waiting around to be done and a good deal of dullness to be endured, they were glad to be taking part in what they felt to be a constructive activity.

But while some patients were willing and even pleased to have students examine them, others were reluctant. 'I ought to start charging for this!' was the standard remark patients on the cardiothoracic wards made as they tacitly agreed to be examined once again, slowly sitting up in bed and undoing the top buttons of their pyjamas to allow students to reach in with their stethoscopes. Taking this joke seriously would raise some interesting questions. Have the patients forgotten their debt to the hospital? Are they hinting that, as taxpayers, they feel entitled to treatment on the National Health Service without having to participate in classes? Perhaps they even feel they should receive payment for allowing their bodies to be used in teaching? But the main point of this remark seems to be to emphasize the frequency with which examinations are requested, and to indicate that they are an inconvenience. This is understandable given that most patients are feeling unwell and are trying to rest. Examinations that involve sitting up and moving, albeit only a little, can become a struggle when a person is in discomfort or is tired.

As the information leaflet suggests (and this is a message which was frequently reiterated by doctors and students themselves), patients were able to say if they preferred not to have medical students involved in their care or did not want to participate in classes. They were told that they would not be treated any differently should they decide to opt out. Some patients did refuse to take part in teaching sessions. Others would avoid them by making excuses, saying that they were expecting visitors or were about to be fetched for tests. In my experience these patients were never made to feel that they had done anything other than exercise their perfect right. At the same time, however, there was a definite expectation among both doctors and students that patients should and would agree to take part in teaching sessions. There was also a definite sense among patients that it was best to agree to any requests doctors and students might make of them in this regard. Refusals might be interpreted as non-compliant behaviour. In the teaching sessions that I observed, then, a particular, historically well-established prerogative was being exercised or enacted by the teaching doctors. Often without being aware of the fact, they were using the leverage of patient debt and obligation to engage patients as teaching material for medical students. Patients' participation, even when offered willingly, can only be understood as semi- or quasi-voluntary in this context. Symptoms, signs and sounds are offered up, partly at least, in recognition of care received or solicited.

'Classic cases'

In the previous chapter I suggested that teaching doctors tended to focus on patients who were of high 'instructive value' (Foucault 1973:59). These patients were usually those thought to exhibit 'good clinical signs', signs that were typical of a particular condition. For example, at one teaching session a patient was used because she presented the 'classic' signs of liver failure. Although we generally looked at cardiology cases under Dr Coltart, he was absent on this particular day and another doctor in his team took charge of the teaching session. She led us to the Intensive Care Unit and over to a woman who was lying in bed, clearly seriously ill. The patient would occasionally make strange crying noises, but she did not move and her eyes were closed. The registrar informed us that the patient was in a coma. Speaking to her in a loud voice but clearly without the expectation of being heard or understood, she said 'Hello, I just want to borrow you for a moment,' and lifted away the sheet that had half covered the woman's body. Looking around at the students, I could see shock and discomfort on all their faces. None of us had seen a person in this condition before. Her abdomen was hugely swollen and distended. The registrar pointed this out with a reflex hammer and said that it was 'a clear sign of liver failure, a type of fluid retention known as "ascites"'. Pointing to the patient's excess facial hair, the registrar said this had grown as a result of hormonal imbalance caused by liver malfunction. She also told us to note the smell in the air caused by the patient's breath (sometimes referred to as 'fetor hepaticus'). She then wanted us all to observe the tremors in the patient's muscles that were characteristic of the condition in its advanced stages. We took it in turns to slide our fingers under those of the patient, which were tightly curled-up, the muscles gripping and relaxing very quickly in a kind of spasm. It was a strange feeling because it was as though the woman was trying to cling to us. We were told, though, this was an involuntary movement. The registrar explained that each of the signs she had pointed out were classic indicators of liver failure in its advanced stages, brought on in this case by chronic alcohol abuse. Once we had left the ward she took us to one side and told us in a low voice that the patient's chance of mortality had been estimated at ninety-nine percent. We were all shaken by the experience of being so close to such a sick patient, and the registrar noticed and dismissed the class. Ironically, we all felt we needed a drink. We washed our hands thoroughly with alcohol and went to the pub.

Of course the medical students were also taught through patients who exhibited less severe symptoms and did not require such intensive management. Each Monday morning, for instance, a firm of students would sit in on Dr Coltart's outpatient clinic, where they usually saw more common and 'everyday' problems than those they tended to meet with on the wards. For instance, they would see patients whose blood pressure needed regular monitoring or whose medications required a review. In the outpatient clinic, too, Dr Coltart was always careful to draw attention to 'classic' signs of particular conditions. For instance, one Monday morning a lady of thirty-four who had Down's syndrome came into the clinic accompanied by her father. After examining the lady, Dr Coltart asked her if it would be all right for us (the medical students and myself) to look at her neck. She and her father both agreed that it would be fine. Forming a line, we each introduced ourselves and looked closely where Dr Coltart had indicated. Once Dr Coltart had told the patient and her father that he felt she was doing nicely and the two had left the room, he explained that he had wanted us to see the flaps of skin around her neck. This was an example of 'webbing', a classic sign of Down's Syndrome. 'You will never see a better example of webbing that that,' he told us. He reiterated that he had shown us so that we would recognize it were we ever to encounter it again.

Patients tended to be selected for teaching, then, when they exhibited good clinical signs. In classes involving auscultation, Dr Coltart would try to select patients with distinctive murmurs for us to listen to. On one of our first teaching sessions on the ward he led us to an elderly female patient from India who, it was rumoured, had come to the hospital suffering from 'Heathrow Syndrome'. This humorous term is used to describe patients who 'happen' to have been taken ill after getting off the plane from a foreign country. These patients often state that they came to Britain to visit relatives. Rather than the illness being a passing 'turn', however, it becomes apparent that a serious operation is needed, which will, since the patient is now in Britain, be carried out and paid for by the NHS. In this particular case it was gathered that as a young woman the patient had married and gone to live in Nigeria for a number of years. There she had suffered a severe fever that was believed by the doctors to have been rheumatic fever. This had damaged her aortic and mitral valves, causing her to suffer valve disease in later life and creating very clearly discernible heart murmurs which Dr Coltart wanted us to listen to.

On another occasion Dr Coltart led us over to a bed in which a young man was sitting. He asked each of us to take a turn examining him, checking his hands to assess the circulation, checking his pulse and so on. Dr Coltart explained that the man was undergoing treatment for heroin addiction and that the tricuspid valve commonly becomes infected in intravenous drug users. The needles are often not sterile, and because users inject into a vein, infected blood returning to the heart meets the tricuspid valve before any of the other valves. The bacteria therefore tend to 'sit on' and infect the tricuspid valve, hampering its function and generating a murmur. When it came to auscultation, Dr Coltart advised that we pay particular attention to the tricuspid area. We were all able to hear a murmur there. Several of us also returned to this man after the teaching session to ask to listen to his murmur once again. Our interest affirmed his status as a source of instruction and a clinical example, but our listening also served to mark out his murmur as a distinct focus of attention.

Medicine and acoustic objectification

During auscultation the diaphragm and/or bell of the stethoscope is applied at designated points that are known to offer the best acoustic perspective on the organ or section of organ beneath. This creates a particular auditory focus on a small part of the body such as a single heart valve. Through an intense auditory concentration, the listener then isolates a particular sound, momentarily excluding other noise coming either from the patient's body or the surrounding environment. Auscultation allows individual sounds to be heard in such a way that they are drawn apart, made the distinct objects of acoustic scrutiny.

Above it was suggested that auditory experience has been characterized as 'intimate, concrete and tactile' (Gell 1995:235). Visual experience, on the other hand, is associated with a detachment and distance that enables the production of discrete perceptual 'objects'. In many ways, auscultation seems to fit this description of auditory experience. The listener and the heart sounds are brought close in perceptual space. The sounds are physically present, their impact upon the ears becoming almost tangible. There is a subtle contact. But at the same time, stethoscopic listening produces a perceptual distance and detachment more commonly associated with visual gazing. It allows the listener to isolate particular sounds, making them discrete. Auscultation, then, creates the possibility of acoustic objectification in the sense that it produces sounds as external and concrete perceptual objects.

Western biomedical practices involve the transformation of the body into frames of reference which create objectification at many levels: 'medico–clinical dehumanization assumes a host of forms, where even living bodies are fragmented and transformed into scientific work objects' (Sharp 2000:298). Indeed, auscultation is one of a range of medical techniques that allow the body to be broken down into its physiological components, its constitutive structures, organs and tissues. As indicated in Chapter 3, Foucault suggests that stethoscopic listening constitutes an auditory complement to, or extension of, a powerful and pervasive visual gaze which is directed in such a way as to make possible ever more extensive examinations of the surface and interior of the human body (1973:164–5). Here, vision and hearing essentially serve the same purpose: isolating and objectifying corporeal details with the aim of broadening and deepening medical knowledge of the body.

Lewis describes how the process of separating out parts of the body and isolating pathologies of disease is essential in enabling people to conceptualize an illness, constructing it as an 'it', an entity (2000:11). He writes: 'in trying to identify or characterize diseases, we select and focus on the signs and symptoms – attributes that people feel or show or that we can find in them' (ibid.). This process constitutes the basis for understanding an illness and for deciding how it should be treated. Lewis, then, suggests that objectification is part of a constructive process of engaging with disease. It is an activity in which both the patient and those addressing the needs of the patient participate. Particular signs or symptoms may become reified, but, argues Lewis, 'that is part of their point and what makes them useful' (ibid.:13). Jackson also observes that some patients find the objectification of their symptoms to be helpful and beneficial, allowing them to establish for themselves, for instance, that the pain they experience is objective and hence 'out-there-and-real' rather than subjective and as a consequence 'not-real' (1994:204).

On one occasion during fieldwork, I encountered a patient who had been suffering from chest pain for several months and had undergone a battery of tests, some of which she had found upsetting and painful, in order to determine the cause. It was only when her case was referred to a particular doctor, whom I had also come to know during fieldwork, that the mystery was solved. The doctor had examined this patient thoroughly and listened to her body carefully, detecting a sound produced as a result of an aortic aneurism, a swelling in the aorta (the aorta is the largest artery in the body, originating from the left ventricle of the heart and extending down into the abdomen). The doctor felt strongly that the abnormality should have been detected by those responsible for the lady's initial examination. Their not having noticed was something of a professional embarrassment. After making her own diagnosis, the doctor suggested the lady listen to her murmur. I asked her why she thought this was a good idea.

> After having so many doctors examine her it would be very rude not to let her listen to herself. It's a mark of dignity for her. She may be thinking 'I have something really wrong with me,' but letting her listen to the murmur and explaining why you were listening may alleviate her worries about other illnesses. In this particular case, I know the patient is intelligent. She has been ill and never known why. Allowing her to listen to her heart lets her say to herself: 'Now I understand why I have been having these symptoms.' She now has something definite to connect her thoughts to. She can hear the sound and understand what's going on. But you have to judge which patients want this kind of knowledge and which don't. Some patients don't want to know or learn about this kind of thing.

Letting this patient use the stethoscope to listen to herself might be interpreted as a considerate but somewhat condescending gesture, a token nod to an illusory equality between doctor and patient. This doctor, however, considered that letting her listen was a way of actively involving the patient in the diagnostic process, sharing it with her and giving her a sense of inclusion. The doctor also hoped that the patient's hearing the murmur might serve as a kind of explanation, the sound declaring the cause and confirming the physiological basis of her suffering. It would be a definite, objective sign that she could recognise and which could become the focus of what had previously been disparate and unfocused anxieties about her health. When I spoke to the patient, she described how she had heard 'a whooshy, gushing sort of sound which shouldn't be there. It made the problem more credible, made me think "Yes, something is going on there."' The murmur was an indication of an underlying problem that she was able to confirm empirically. This lady also said that she felt being offered the chance to listen to her own murmur constituted an important mark of respect. 'It's like they're saying "We're all listening to you, maybe you should hear what's going on." It made me feel more like a person, less like a chunk of meat.' The doctor's decision to let the patient listen to herself had obviously been a good one.

In this case the patient as well as the doctor is able to isolate and objectify the murmur through listening. Auto-auscultation permits a kind of auto-objectification. In her study of chronic pain sufferers, Jackson (1994) observes that patients frequently objectify their own pain symptoms or affected body parts. She suggests that this represents a common and generally constructive step in patients' efforts to distance themselves from their pain, allowing them to manage it more effectively. For the patient introduced above, too, auto-objectification is a productive and positive act.

On the cardiothoracic wards where my research at St Thomas' took place, doctors to whom I spoke acknowledged that it was often difficult to explain in detail to patients what a heart murmur was without that explanation creating additional fear and concern. The best thing, it was felt, was to tell the patient that he or she had a murmur in the heart and that this meant one of the valves was leaking slightly. To say more or to suggest that the patient listen to the murmur would mean going into more and more medical specifics which would have to be explained, making the patient's understanding of the problem increasingly complex and, in all likelihood, confused. It was felt that listening to a murmur, while not necessarily a bad idea for patients who were particularly intelligent, engaged and calm, would usually only exacerbate anxiety. As a result, it was unusual for patients to be given the opportunity to listen to their own heart murmurs. The doctor in the example above recognized that it was the patient's intelligence, and the necessity of an especially attentive gesture following the incompetence displayed so far in her treatment, that made it sensible for her to listen to the sound in question. In general, though, it was preferable for the stethoscope, and the diagnostic perspective it both represents and enables, to remain in the hands of the doctor. I describe below how patients who had consented to repeated auscultation through being involved in the training of medical students were frequently uncomfortable with the way in which their murmurs had seemingly become separated from the 'synergistic interplay' through which they experienced their bodies (Taussig 1992:96). Rather than feeling involved or included in the diagnostic process, they often felt themselves to have been reduced to objects of clinical interest, 'things' to be listened to.

Auscultation and 'dehumanization'

It was explained above that in the teaching and learning of auscultation, patients with 'good' murmurs tended to attract considerable attention. Doctors sometimes referred to such patients metonymically as, for instance, 'the beautiful aortic stenosis is bed nineteen' or 'the wonderful mitral regurgitation in bed six'. There is clearly already a type of clinical objectification taking place here, patients being identified through their diagnostic signs rather than by their names or other non-medical attributes.

Patients with exemplary murmurs were also sometimes referred to as 'celebrity' patients because of the amount of attention they received. 'I've been examined by thirty-six medical students today!' one man responded when I asked him if many people had asked to listen to his chest. This was an unusually high number but it was common for a patient with good clinical signs to be visited by two or three groups of perhaps seven or eight medical students, accompanied by teaching doctors, in a single day. While patients were selected because of their exemplary heart sounds, teaching doctors also gave thought as to which patients would be easiest or best to listen to, observing, for instance, whether or not patients were overweight, as the heart sounds can be muffled by subcutaneous fat. Thin patients were preferred, young men being ideal as they tend to have very little fat or breast tissue. During classes patients would be asked to assume particular positions, lying down, sitting up at forty-five degrees or sitting forward so as to give doctors and students the optimum chance of hearing and identifying abnormal sounds. They would be requested to take deep breaths in order to maximize blood and air flow to parts of the heart and lungs. Rather like grand pianos being set up for a concert, patients were positioned so as to produce the best possible acoustic.

On one occasion I was speaking to a 'celebrity patient' when our conversation was interrupted by a group of students under the instruction of a senior doctor. The students were practising for their fourth-year medical exams and their teacher wanted them to listen to the patient's heart, which produced the murmur of mitral stenosis. I went into the adjoining room while the students carried out their examination. When they had finished I returned, and asked the patient how he felt about being examined by so many people. He replied that he did not enjoy feeling like an 'object of special interest' particularly. 'It's only happened because the sound's a bit loud or a bit different, or funnier than normal', he said. He had become conscious of his status as a kind of acoustic exhibit.

Other patients reacted similarly to repeated auscultation. They related feeling like 'containers' or 'showcases' for the clinical signs in which the medics were interested. One woman said she felt her heart had become like a tape recorder, playing the same sound for all the people who came to listen. It was the murmur, rather than any of the other details of her case that they wanted to hear. Others were visibly tired of repeated examinations. When students requested 'a little listen' they would roll their eyes or wordlessly hold open their gowns so that the students could get to the necessary points of the chest. One patient described how it was almost as if the process were 'nothing to do with' her. As far as she was concerned the students were solely intent upon listening to her murmur.

Asked how she felt about receiving so many listening visitors, one 'celebrity' patient replied:

> At the moment I am quite relaxed about it, but in general I do feel it to be an invasion of privacy. It's dehumanizing. It can make you feel like you're a leaf under a microscope. There's no bond. It's just anonymous people listening to something that's going on in your body. They see you as a kind of clinical curiosity. As I say, I'm quite relaxed about it now, but I have taken exception to it at other times in my life. You may be helping by refining medical students but it is certainly not fulfilling for you as a patient. It's a clinical and anonymous process. It's rude. It's invasive, though, right now, as I say, I'm quite relaxed about it.

This patient explained that she appreciated doctors taking the time to listen carefully to her body and described herself as 'grateful to the stethoscope' for the light that it had thrown on her condition. She had, however, spent some time in hospital and was beginning to take exception to the repeated examinations that she was undergoing. A number of medical students to whom I spoke were also aware that when listening to hearts there was a tendency to encounter a patient simply as a set of acoustic signs. As Tom remarked, 'Sometimes I become really conscious that all we do is reduce people to two heart sounds and a murmur.' He pointed out that just as the stethoscope was in essence a small amplifier, it had the effect of amplifying the heart sounds in such a way that they came to drown out other considerations, eventually eclipsing 'the patient' altogether.

It is important to state that some people enjoyed being celebrity patients. One, for instance, had learned the technical term for his murmur over the course of several examinations. He liked being able to test the students when they came to visit him. Others also enjoyed the chance to interact with the students, who usually took great care to be polite, friendly and good-humoured. But while some patients appreciated the contact that the teaching interaction generated, most felt their bodies to have become objectified as acoustic curiosities. Their wider qualities, characteristics and concerns were disregarded. Here auscultation sets up a doctor-patient relationship from which, paradoxically, many patients felt themselves to be curiously absent. In Chapter 3 it was explained that the emergence of auscultation allowed doctors to attend less to patients' narrations of their illnesses and to focus instead on sounds as empirically verifiable diagnostic signs. Perhaps, even at an early stage in the development of the technique, there was an intimation that auscultation might create situations in which doctors overlooked the disease and patient in a holistic sense, devoting themselves instead to an intense focus on sounds as diagnostic signs.

Auscultation and sexual objectification

One of the reasons Rene Laennec initially objected to immediate auscultation was that for a Frenchman in the early nineteenth century, pressing an ear to the chest of a young female involved an unacceptable level of intimacy. The stethoscope was created partly as a way of preserving decency, allowing the doctor to remove himself to a socially acceptable distance. But using the stethoscope still requires the doctor to be close, within what we might consider the patient's 'personal space'. Mediate auscultation also requires intimate contact in that the diaphragm of the stethoscope, if not the doctor's ear, is applied to the patient's chest. At the same time, although it is sometimes possible to listen through thin layers of clothing, the technique works best when the stethoscope is placed directly on the skin and the location of the best listening points means that the patient may be required to remove at least some clothes on the top half of his or her body. Auscultation therefore necessitates a degree of physical exposure.

Though in medical terms a 'non-invasive' examination (and it is certainly much less invasive than many other diagnostic procedures), some female patients in particular did not experience auscultation as such. In classes, Dr Coltart would give us tacit instruction on how to manage the awkwardness created by the invasion of privacy that the technique involves. During outpatient consultations he would slip the diaphragm of the stethoscope under the shirts of female patients to save them having to do anything more than undo a few buttons, indicating that we might do the same as we became more competent listeners. Patients on the ward tended to be in bed wearing only gowns or pyjamas, and sometimes nothing at all, so that there examinations usually involved more exposure on the part of the patient. Students copied the way Dr Coltart focused on a point beyond the patient or allowed his eyes to close or take on an absent expression. This was helpful not only as a way of aiding auditory concentration, but also in serving to restrict or divert a wandering and potentially offensive gaze. It drew attention away from, rather than towards the patient, making his or her exposure less obvious and acute.

Though it was important to manage the intimacy of stethoscopic listening in a serious and professional manner in interactions with patients, that same intimacy sometimes became the subject of humour. One patient told the students how much he liked it when pretty young female medical students came to examine him. He laughed as he described the way they fawned over his chest, but insisted that they loved it even more than he did. Humour around auscultation was particularly pronounced in 'backstage' contexts. 'Look, I'm doing you a huge favour, cardiology will do wonders for your relationship,' Dr Coltart told the students one day, trying to galvanize their interest in auscultation. He said that when they got home they should get their partners to take their shirts off and lie down on the sofa, then practise listening to their chests. 'It's the perfect seduction technique!' The students laughed a lot at this. They laughed, too, when two of their group, rumoured to be romantically connected, were caught listening to each other's hearts in a bay off one of the hospital corridors.

In Western culture the heart is often considered the seat of love and desire. A poem by Lorca nicely captures a romantically inflected auscultatory act, the poet describing how a lover 'wants to press his ear to the sleeping girl and understand the Morse code of her heart...' (Lorca 1928, cited Maurer 2001:xviii). In a similar way, a medical student told me one day that he would be taking his 'emotional stethoscope' with him when he went to see a particular girl friend of his, as he could not tell whether or not she had feelings for him. When I looked confused he explained that the stethoscope was, after all, 'a device for listening to hearts'. But while auscultation is a useful metaphor for attempting to discern the secrets of the heart as the affective core, the technique is also potentially sexually charged through the particular sensuality it creates. As indicated in Chapter 5, as well as entailing the at least partial exposure of the patient's chest to sight and touch, the participants are brought close enough to be able to feel the warmth of one another. They can hear and feel each other's breathing. They can smell one another. When the interaction involves physical attraction, this intimacy can take on clear erotic overtones. A good illustration of the sexual frisson created by (in this case immediate) auscultation is highlighted in Mike Newell's (2007) film of Marquez's (1989) *Love in the Time of Cholera*, when a young and handsome Dr Juvenal Urbino first encounters his future wife, the beautiful Fermina Daza. She has a fever and he examines her by pressing an ear to her bare chest.

During fieldwork, some students talked about a website which boasted 'stethoscope porn'. They didn't say that they enjoyed it, but rather they were astonished by its freakishness. *Heartbeat Babes* advertised itself as a 'heartbeat and stethoscope fetish' site. The general term for this kind of material is apparently 'cardiorotica', which involves the eroticization of medical equipment, diagnostic techniques and interactions relating to the heart. At the time of writing the homepage of *Heartbeat Babes* boasted a large image of a topless woman in white high heels, stockings, knickers and a nurse's hat, sitting on a table and leaning back whilst smiling at the viewer. Sensors and cables of the kind used for electrocardiograms were fitted to her naked torso and connected to a monitor. There were also smaller images of semi-naked women making themselves available for auscultation and other chest examinations, while one showed a woman holding open her shirt and listening to her own heart with a stethoscope. I did not explore the site any further than accessing the homepage. These images, however, knowingly allude to and consciously exaggerate the visual and tactile intimacy created by the stethoscopic interaction and other techniques of cardiological investigation. They invite the viewer to dwell on the erotic potential of auscultation and to fantasize about being involved in explicitly sexualized stethoscopic interactions.

As well as showing images of auscultation, the homepage draws attention to the erotic thrill of hearing women's heartbeats. The point of the site seems to be not just to enable users to look at the women depicted, but to listen to them. 'Watch videos where you can actually hear the sound of the girls [sic] heartbeats as they ride bikes, do sit ups and star jumps,' urges the text. 'If you're into stethoscopes, heartbeats, stress tests or blood pressure cuffs then this is the site for you!' It asks the visitor: 'where else can you watch real live videos of girls being stethed and hear their heartbeat pounding away?' Also advertized are downloadable recordings of heartbeats. Comments from (very probably fictional) *Heartbeat Babes* 'fans' include:

> The latest Anna and Yvonne shoot is just too good for words. Your exercise bike videos are incredible! Anna stething Yvonne just after she does that bike is one for the Heartbeat Hall-of-Fame! The sound of her heart pounding is incredible and I like the fact that we get to listen to it until after it goes back to resting, nice job!'
>
> I've never seen anything so erotic as these two ladies auscultating each other. I love the differences in their hearts: Anna's is always slow, around 60, not exceeding 142 after exercise, matching her persona: wise, sleepy, sexy in a knowing way. Yvonne's is quicker, more nervous, around 72 at rest, zooming to over 180 after exercise. Her sweet, innocent, madonna-like face while being auscultated, her dark hair spread over the pillow, is a huge turn on.
>
> Hats off to you for developing this new site. It certainly is what we who love a woman's heartbeat have wanted for a long time.

The 'visitors,' then, make reference to the visual images and express pleasure in watching scenes of auscultation and cardiac investigation. But they also declare a very specific kind of acousticophilia or sexual arousal derived from sounds. Though most commonly associated with music, here the term can be understood to index a particular, fetishized interest in listening to heartbeats, an idea I explore in more detail through a piece of short fiction that is included as the appendix of this book (Rice 2008b). The comments reference a kind of auditory jouissance, an 'ecstasy of hearing', an intense erotic appreciation of the qualities of the heartbeat and the patterns of the heart rate which the women on the site are effectively modelling (Ingold 2000:271).

Jordanova (1989) explores the phenomenon of dissection as the key technique used to expand medical knowledge of the body in the late eighteenth and early nineteenth centuries. She argues that medicine at this time was preoccupied with explaining the differences between the male and the female body. Medicine was an almost exclusively male profession and dissections most often involved the body of a woman. The numerous anatomical wax models made in this period were also generally female and, Jordanova writes, positioned 'in passive, yet sexually inviting poses' (ibid.:42). These figures, she suggests, were knowingly erotic: 'the viewer was intended to respond to the model as to a female body that delighted the sight and invited sexual thoughts' (ibid.:55). Scophilia, 'the drive to look', and epistemophilia, 'the desire to know', became fused in erotically nuanced practices of medical gazing (Grosz 1992:447).

The stethoscope fetish has arguably originated from, or at least may be associated with, the sexualized thread within medical knowledge practices that Jordanova identifies. The images of women connected to medical machines or undergoing examinations, and the recordings of heart sounds on *Heartbeat Babes,* seem to imply a voyeuristic engagement with a simultaneously sexualized and medically scrutinized, if not anatomized, female body. Also, although it is no longer an exclusively male profession, medicine in the West has traditionally been male-dominated so that auscultation can be positioned as a gendered activity, closely associated with male knowledge and power.

As a website, use of *Heartbeat Babes* is not restricted to people of a specific gender or sexual orientation. However, the visual content of the homepage seems to be primarily orientated towards heterosexual men. The comments cited above also adopt a heterosexual and distinctly male voice. Although it does not preclude enjoyment by women, both the style and content of the site seem directed toward a pornographic convention in which women are displayed or exhibited as sexual objects for the stimulation and enjoyment of males. Several authors draw attention to the role of visual gazing in the positioning of women as sexual objects. A classic example is Mulvey's (1975) discussion of cinema as an apparatus for the production of male sexual pleasure and power derived from the visual objectification of women. In a similar way, Berger (1972) suggests that the nude as a genre of painting involves a politics of vision through which women are presented as sexual objects and male possessions. In *Heartbeat Babes* it is partly through a process of acoustic objectification that women are situated as sexualized beings-for-men. Indeed, rather than being light-heartedly dismissed as an unusual form of sex toy, the stethoscope might be interpreted as an instrument that diversifies and augments the male gaze and its colonization of the female body.

Schafer states that '[t]he ear is an erotic orifice. Listening to beautiful sounds, for instance the sounds of music, is like the tongue of a lover in your ear' (1977:11–12). The erotic potential of auditory experience is linked to the ear's receptivity (arguably lending the ear a feminized sexual identity). But listening can also be an active means of inquiry, and in stethoscopic listening the metaphorical shape of the ear is reversed so that it becomes an active, penetrating proboscis. In the context of *Heartbeat Babes* it becomes a kind of surrogate penis, enabling the acoustic penetration of female bodies. At the same time, auscultation initiates and provides context for both the undressing of the women on display and the particular poses they adopt. The technique is used to frame the doctor-patient interaction as a form of association characterized by an always latent, and sometimes overt, erotic charge.

De-fetishizing the stethoscope

It might be argued that this book is itself an expression of a kind of stethoscope fetish. It seems to be the product of an excessive or irrational interest in auscultation and techniques of medical listening. At the same time the book might be accused of fetishizing the stethoscope by assigning it seemingly magical powers to shape sensory activity and experience, declare ideological shifts and mediate human relationships. Indeed, Chapter 4 explored contexts in which the stethoscope might be understood to possess agency in its own right. But the instrument cannot be considered to produce patterns of thought and action in a predictable or deterministic fashion through some power of its own. As the *Heartbeat Babes* website ably demonstrates, any functions and meanings which the stethoscope is brought to serve and articulate are heavily dependent upon the context of its use and the intentions of its users.

Sharp (2000) points out that medical work has involved the systematic objectification of the body and its parts and processes. However, as we have seen, value judgments should not be attached to objectification *per se*. It may be understood as an important perceptual stage in the production of medical knowledge and in the conceptualization of diseases and their pathology. Also, as Lewis (2000) and Jackson (1994) point out, objectification is a valuable conceptual step in the structuring of illness experience and can be helpful in organizing responses to symptoms. However, through auscultation in medical student training, particularly when repeated listening is practised, patients can become acutely conscious of their being positioned as acoustic beings-for-others rather than beings-for-themselves. This tendency of repeated stethoscopic listening to objectify patients in negatively experienced ways can be used to discredit the notion that hearing is somehow an intrinsically positive, receptive and benevolent sense, inherently productive of sympathy and inclusivity. The voices of patients suggest otherwise.

At a practical level, the chapter indicates that there may be real benefits in doctors and medical students being sensitive to the impacts that diagnostic processes, however seemingly gentle and familiar, can have on their patients. The careful and considerate action of the doctor described above who allowed a patient to listen to the sound made by her own aortic aneurism shows that negatively experienced forms of medical objectification can be circumvented or counterbalanced through good management, which in this particular case involved taking steps to make auscultation an inclusive rather than an exclusive acoustic practice. The chapter also shows that processes of acoustic objectification may take a range of forms, and may in certain medical contexts be multi-layered, multi-faceted and intense. Types of acoustic objectification also point to different types of doctor-patient relationship, or, more accurately, highlight some of the different aspects of or potentials within doctor-patient interactions. In doing so they remind us of a particular set of knowledge, power and gender relations that have historically underpinned and continue to inform doctor-patient relationships within Western medicine.

This chapter draws on material from Tom Rice, '"Beautiful murmurs": stethoscopic listening and acoustic objectification', published in *Senses & Society* 3(3):293–306. Reproduced with permission.

CHAPTER 7

Auto-auscultation

Listening to the Self

The previous chapter made reference to an instance of auto-auscultation in which a woman was invited to listen to herself using a stethoscope. This chapter explores the phenomenon of auto-auscultation more closely. Firstly, it describes how medical students are encouraged to listen to themselves in order to develop a sense of what 'normal' heart sounds are like and to acquire familiarity with the cardiac cycle. Auscultation is a skill that is best practised by listening to an actual person, and for the students, listening to themselves was a way of learning to listen to others. Secondly, it examines situations in which sounds produced through auscultation, but also electrocardiography and echocardiography, bring patients to engage with their own interiority, a form of listening that often provokes anxiety. Thirdly, it introduces a form of auto-auscultation in which patients' heart sounds are so loud as to be audible to them without a stethoscope, creating what can be disturbing experiences. In each of these situations, auto-auscultation produces an acoustic engagement not with 'the body' in an abstract sense, but with the person's own body, the 'my body', the body as it belongs to and is experienced by the subject (Sawday 1995).

In a series of reflections on sound that amount to a critique of the term 'soundscape', Ingold draws parallels with ideas put forward in his work on the weather (2006, 2007a). He points out that the medium of sound is generally the air, and that the air is in a continual state of movement and flux; the everyday term for these fluxes is 'the weather'. Anthropologists working on sound should, Ingold suggests, increase their attention to the medium of sound and as a result, 'our metaphors for describing auditory space should', he argues, 'be derived not from landscape studies but from meteorology' (2006).

Ingold goes on to note that there is a tendency in academic discussions to refer to the 'embodied experience' of the weather, as if the weather somehow undergoes a process of consolidation in and through bodily experience. But, he suggests, given that a person may be, for instance, buffeted about, cooled or warmed by a strong breeze, it would be more accurate to say that it is not the wind that is embodied but the person that is 'en-winded' (ibid.). In a similar way, Ingold argues, sound moves through the air, cocooning, sweeping past and flowing around the listener. So in auditory experience too it is not sound that is embodied but the body that is 'ensounded' (ibid.). Ingold works from the premise that sounds are always external, surrounding and enveloping the listener. But sounds are also produced internally. They originate within and are conducted through the substance of the body: through tissue and blood. 'Sound inhabits the subject just as the subject might be said to inhabit sound' (Bull 2000:2). The concept of 'ensoundedness' must be expanded, then, to include not only a listener's dwelling in sound, but also sound dwelling in the listener.

Psycho-acousticians have for a long time recognized a range of internally generated sounds produced by the movement of the organs, tissues and fluid inside the body (Barany 1938, Tonndorf 1972). Human bodies, like the bodies of other organisms, are 'hives of activity, pulsing with the flows of materials that keep them alive' (Ingold 2007b:12). They are collections of happenings, some of which produce sounds. To me, the notion of the body as a 'hive of activity' conjures up images of a hive of bees, forming one large organism, constantly active and engaged in innumerable tiny tasks and processes, giving off a distinctive buzzing sound. The body can be conceptualized in a similar way, not as a static entity but as a multitude of movements and happenings that also produce sounds.

In his discussion of reggae sound systems, Henriques introduces the concept of the 'sonic body' (2003:471). He writes that the term 'implies either and both the body of the sound and the sound of the body' (ibid.:471–2). He analyses the experience (simultaneously auditory, tactile, kinaesthetic, erotic and ethnically marked) that is produced in dancers' bodies during the reggae sound system session. The present chapter is more concerned with elements of the 'sound of the body' than the 'body of sound', the latter of which I take to imply the materiality, weight and physical power of the output of the sound system. It focuses on sounds that originate in and are produced by physiological events within the body itself. I consider not so much the embodied experience of sound, as the experience of embodied sound.

Henriques also remarks that 'listening puts us both inside ourselves and outside ourselves' (ibid.:472). This might be interpreted as meaning that a consideration of auditory experience involves both attending to sound in the world and exploring its embodied 'effects and affects' (ibid.:453). Chapter 2 of this book explored how, in the setting of the cardiothoracic unit, sounds complicate ideas of corporeal interiority and exteriority. In this chapter, auto-auscultation provides an additional context in which attending to sound makes a challenge of any differentiation between senses of being 'inside' and 'outside'. It creates a situation, also implied by Henriques, in which listening puts us inside ourselves and outside ourselves simultaneously.

Developing the notion that sounds might be involved in corporeal awareness and a sense of the body-as-self, I draw on Duden's interpretation of the concept of 'hexis', which she defines as 'the habitual state in which a person finds him or herself' (1993:91). I argue that sounds are intertwined with those physical and affective sensations that inform everyday consciousness of the body and its condition. In the case of heart sounds in particular, these are normally quiet, barely if at all at the level of conscious awareness. Auto-auscultation, however, produces situations in which these are brought to the fore, amplified, made distinct; they stand out as elements within the body hexis. The chapter goes on to give examples, recorded in medical literature, of patients who have heart murmurs or abnormal heart sounds so loud they can be heard across a room. While I did not encounter cases quite this severe during fieldwork, some patients I met did experience loud, abnormal sounds emanating from within their own bodies. These could be particularly unpleasant and frightening. Drawing on Leder, I suggest that these disturbing sonic happenings are instances of 'dys-appearance', the 'unwanted consciousness' of one's body that occurs at times of disease or distress and which can produce in a person a sense of alienation from his or her own body (Leder 1990:69, Csordas 1994:8). Even if not immediately associated with other specific physical symptoms, the sounds are likely to be regarded as inconsistent with a normal, healthy body hexis, so becoming a source of serious anxiety and concern. The chapter suggests, then, that heart murmurs *as sounds* can become involved in immediate corporeal experiences of 'feeling' and 'being' unwell.

Social context invariably shapes the interpretation of sound. Henriques explains that in the instance of the reggae sound system, a context is provided which frames the expression and enactment of ecstasy, abandon and intoxication as acceptable, even expected responses to the music. This context makes the sonic body as described by Henriques a very different one from that outlined here. In the hospital, activities unfolded within an environment organized around medical practice. In the case of auto-auscultation, heart sounds (even healthy ones) were identified and interpreted through a framework of medical knowledge. People entering the hospital as patients generally did so against a backdrop of illness or medical concern.

It is unsurprising, then, that auto-auscultation often aggravated feelings of vulnerability, uncertainty and powerlessness that in many cases already accompanied the patient role.

The auscultation of everyone

Dr Coltart told his students that they should listen to people's chests at every available opportunity. This meant not just hospital patients, but people everywhere. He joked that even when we were sitting on the Tube (London's underground transport system) we should ask the person sitting next to us if it would be all right to listen to his or her heart. From many of its rooms St Thomas' Hospital has remarkable views out over the River Thames, the Houses of Parliament and Westminster Bridge. On one occasion Dr Coltart made a sweeping gesture towards the bridge and asked us to imagine what would happen if we were to stop all the people walking across it and listen to their hearts: 'Think of all those interesting sounds. There would be hundreds of people walking around with murmurs who didn't even realize they had them!'

The group would often kill time between teaching sessions drinking coffee in the hospital café. After this session we began to discuss how strange Dr Coltart's idea was. Tom explained:

> You suddenly realize that they are inside everyone, these heart sounds... and the stethoscope is like a window to that. If I just walked around the street and listened to everyone... I would be bound to hear murmurs that people never knew they had, and suddenly they've got a disease, suddenly there's something wrong with them.

Harjit thought similarly: 'I had never really thought about people in that way before. I could go around with my stethoscope and I would pick up heart murmurs in people everywhere, not just in the hospital but in the street.' Making the population at large subject to (albeit hypothetical) medical scrutiny, the students effectively collapsed any distinction between patients and non-patients. They adopted a kind of stethoscopic macro-focus, reminiscent of the project of 'surveillance medicine', whereby entire populations become subject to clinical observation (Armstrong 1995:397).

A student named Dave described how, listening to a CD of heart murmurs as he travelled to the hospital by bus, he was surprised to find himself imposing the murmurs he was hearing onto people he saw in the street as if their (unhealthy) heart sounds were amplified or, having acquired an extraordinary auditory acuity, he could hear them clearly from a distance. The recordings also gave him the feeling that he was auscultating the city, or that the city was producing murmurs so that flows of traffic and people through the streets resembled flows of blood through the vessels and chambers of the heart (see Sennett 1996:263–5). Points of congestion brought to mind malfunctioning valves, and, through Dave's aestheticized 'auditory looking' (where his gaze was influenced by the mediated sounds to which he was listening), they came to represent the ill health of the city itself (Bull 2000:191). Dave's comments could be understood to resonate with a widely held notion that congested and noisy streets are antithetical to an urban ideal where the movement of traffic is smooth and quietly rhythmical, like a healthy heart (Bijsterveld 2003).

Good explores the manner in which Harvard Medical School students are led to 'think anatomically' through their training and as a consequence internalize 'an alternative way of seeing' (1994:73). He suggests that the students carry and apply the gaze they acquire at medical school beyond the campus. After conducting dissections and autopsies, for instance, they begin mentally to anatomize the living people they encounter in everyday life. Good, who conducted participant observation with the students, observes this occurring in himself too:

> While participating in anatomy as an observer, I would occasionally be walking along a street and find myself a body amidst bodies, rather than a person amid persons. I found myself attending to the anatomical features of persons I passed, rather than perceiving them as persons with social characteristics or imagined lives. (ibid.)

Good cites a medical student studying on a module in pathology: 'I'll find myself in a conversation…I'll all of a sudden start to think about, you know, if I took the scalpel and made a cut [on you] right here, what would that look like?' (ibid.). Similarly, the students with whom I studied found their acquired gaze, and in this instance their acoustic perspective on the body, applying beyond the hospital.

Dr Coltart encouraged his students to practise listening on the people close to them as well as people in and outside the hospital. He said they should auscultate their boyfriends and girlfriends but also advised them to listen to their family members. Rather than being applied solely in the context of medical training, this brought the stethoscopic focus to a domestic, familial level. The change proved worrying and difficult. There was always a possibility that the students might hear something they didn't want to. As Mary explained:

> When you're in hospital you want to hear murmurs. You want to hear loads of noises. But I was listening to my Dad's chest and I was thinking 'Please,

> let there be just normal heart sounds, no murmurs.' I was worried because I know he smokes. And I was thinking 'Come on Dad! Be normal! Be normal!' Then I was listening and I thought 'Thank God I can't hear anything! Thank God there are no murmurs.'

Rishi told me about the time he and his identical twin brother who (as explained in Chapter 4) was also studying medicine in the same year, listened to their father's chest:

> I remember my brother listening to my Dad's chest. He's had an MI (Myocardial Infarction or 'heart attack') in '95. Anyway, my brother was listening to my Dad's chest and he heard a diastolic murmur. I came in to the room and I listened and heard it too. My brother and me both agreed it was a diastolic murmur. It worried my Dad – enough to make him go to the GP.

Several other students found their family members were unwilling to undergo the examination at all; they were too concerned about what the stethoscope might reveal. The students disliked momentarily reformulating kinship relationships as doctor-patient relationships, and found they could not maintain the position of distance and detachment that characterized their interactions with the people they saw during teaching sessions.

Sinclair writes that the medical students he studied were told 'Don't listen to your own heart; it's confusing!' (1997:203). However, Dr Coltart actively encouraged us to listen to ourselves. He said it would give us a chance to familiarize ourselves with normal heart sounds (assuming our bodies would be clinically normal and implicitly reaffirming the notion that the doctor should be 'healthy' relative to the 'sick' patient), and would enable us to think through the relationship of the heart sounds to the cardiac cycle. As we ourselves were even more readily available for practice than patients, it made sense to listen to our own hearts.

But bringing a stethoscopic focus to oneself could be frightening; as Tom put it 'You just never know what you're going to hear.' He continued: 'My Dad has had a few heart problems and I'm a bit of a hypochondriac... I don't really want to turn this ear that I'm being trained to use on myself.' In fact, both Tom and Alistair found they had quite bad sinus arrhythmia. This condition can often be observed in young men: the heart tends to speed up perceptibly during inspiration, slowing down again during expiration. Although not a sign of disease or abnormality it can be disconcerting, particularly if an entirely regular heart rhythm is expected. Harjit experienced a similar fear of what she might hear: 'I came back from class and was sitting at my desk and I thought "Wait, I've never listened to my heart before." I was uncertain about whether I should or not. I was very scared that I might hear something bad.' None of the students I studied with detected an abnormality, though it later became known that a medical student in a different firm had heard a murmur and become very distressed. She had gone crying to her teaching doctor and had never been entirely convinced by his reassurances that hers was a 'flow murmur' and therefore 'innocent'. It is easy to understand why she was reluctant to believe him given the strong emphasis placed on murmurs as indicators of valve disease in the medical students' training.

For those who heard their heart sounds as normal, auto-auscultation became a reassuring, even pleasant experience. Some students would try running on the spot while listening to themselves, seeing how fast they could make their hearts beat and how loud they could make them sound. Rishi's friend Ambrose said that he would spend large amounts of time listening to his own heartbeat and would lie in bed, sometimes falling asleep with the stethoscope still in his ears. He found the experience comforting and speculated that this might be because auscultation created acoustic conditions similar to those inside the womb. His suggestion chimes with the notion that the environment in which the foetus develops is sonically rich, the heartbeat of the mother being a distinctive rhythmic presence, a 'steady clarion of safety' (Murch 1994:vii, DeNora 2000:77, Ackerman 1990:178–9, [quotation Ackerman 1990:179]).

It is clear, then, that diagnostic techniques and the perspectives they create do not remain restricted to the hospital setting. Instead, they spill out of the clinical context, creating informal perceptual engagements and interactions. Students encounter not only 'the body', unassociated with a specific owner or linked to a socially distant patient, but also socially close and familiar bodies through medical schemes of perception. Turning the stethoscope back on themselves they also encounter their own lived and experienced bodies – what Draper (2002) calls the 'my body' – in new and potentially unsettling ways.

Patients as listeners

Normally there is a clear distinction between the person who listens with the stethoscope (generally the doctor or medical student), and the person who is listened to (the patient). When students become their own practice patients, however, this distinction becomes blurred. 'Listener' and 'listened-to' are the same person. This is also true in situations where patients listen to themselves. As explained in the previous chapter, few patients are given the opportunity to listen to their own hearts using a stethoscope. Doctors told me that this was because auto-auscultation would be likely to generate more confusion and anxiety on the part of patients than it would resolve. Although in the case of auto-auscultation mentioned in the previous chapter the patient benefited from listening to herself (whilst carefully directed by the doctor in charge of her care), there was a general sense among doctors that most patients did not want to know what was going on inside their own bodies. As Sawday indicates, people often have an aversion to engaging with their own interiority (1995:15). This sentiment was expressed by several of the patients to whom I spoke. One man explained: 'I don't mind what the doctors do, where they poke or prod, as long as I don't have to know what is going on inside me or what the surgeon is actually going to do when he comes to operate.' He said that thinking about his heart or imagining it in any way made him feel 'queasy'.

An example of the discomfort that could be created by a patient listening directly to his own heart was provided when one morning during a teaching session we were ushered to the bed of a sixty-five year old Turkish man. Dr Coltart introduced us all to him and we spent some minutes practising our cardio-respiratory examination, paying particular attention to the man's murmur. That afternoon I accompanied a student who went back to listen to the murmur again and the man and I began to talk about his stay in hospital. He explained that he had been aware since he was in his twenties that he had a problem with his heart. At that time a doctor had told him he had a murmur and explained about the leaking mitral valve it indicated. However, the doctor had apparently decided not to intervene as the problem was not serious. 'After all, I didn't need to be an Olympic athlete, I just needed to lead a normal life,' the man explained. He was in no pain and had lived generally very comfortably until three days earlier when he had collapsed and been taken to hospital in Sidcup, Kent. There it was found that his mitral valve had prolapsed. He had been transferred to St Thomas' where doctors were deciding whether to replace his mitral valve or repair the existing one.

At this point, the man began to tell me about a friend of his who was a cardiologist in Turkey. They had met at university where the friend had studied medicine. Some years ago, this same friend had presented him with a stethoscope as a gift and said: 'Listen to yourself from time to time.' The man had thought the present a strange one, but told his friend that it would act as a reminder of his murmur and of the fact that he should look after himself. The friend taught him to press the stethoscope to his side in order to hear the murmur best and told the man that he should see a doctor if the sound got louder or changed dramatically. 'So I listened to myself from time to time. But I didn't like the noise. The heart is irregular and it has a loud noise in it.' He began to cry, and said through his tears, 'The listening filled me with disquiet.' Clearly this man had experienced his heart murmur as a disturbing presence, an unwelcome reminder of his lingering medical problem. He also experienced the murmur as an aesthetically unpleasant noise, by association sinister and threatening.

As indicated in Chapters 1 and 2, the tones of ECG or electrocardiograph machines were almost constantly audible on the cardiothoracic wards where I conducted fieldwork. Some patients recognized these tones as a sonic representation of their heartbeats, meaning that listening to them produced an experience of a kind of auto-auscultation. A few patients remarked that they liked being able to hear their own hearts beating away and found it reassuring. But more felt that it was frightening. Suffering from heart problems as they were, they preferred not to think about what was going on inside their bodies at all. As one man explained: 'I know somebody has to know about my heart, but I'd just rather not and this way I have to.' He didn't like the auditory reminder of his vulnerability that the electrocardiograph produced. 'It sometimes sounds to me like the thing is counting down,' said a patient named Colin. 'You don't know how many pips you've got left.' 'When it's you connected up you're always waiting for the next beep, worrying that it's not going to come,' added his ward neighbour. For these patients the electrocardiograph reinforced a sense of their lives being in jeopardy. Medical dramas and films with emergency room resuscitation scenes, of course, exploit this quality of the electrocardiograph's beep. The action often culminates in a spell of silence with the sudden resumption of the beep signifying a life narrowly saved. Alternatively there is also the now rather clichéd continuous tone or 'flat line,' indicating death (though cardiologists I have spoken to assure me that this tone is never actually heard, as a stopped heart produces no beat and therefore no tone at all).

As with electrocardiography, patients' experiences of the sounds produced during echocardiography could also constitute a kind of auto-auscultation. For instance, one young man I spoke to was in hospital for an infection that had damaged the mitral valve of his heart. He took the sounds produced during the echocardiogram to be an amplification of a murmur made by his blood as it leaked through the damaged valve (he had heard the doctors referring to this 'murmur' during previous examinations). 'It sounded pretty loud,' he told me. 'I'm glad they've decided to do something about it' (by which he meant operate and replace the valve). An elderly lady I spoke to on several occasions had received a number of echocardiograms over the years in order to monitor a leak in her aortic valve. 'On the echo you can actually hear it and it's not very nice,' she said. 'You can actually hear what's going on inside your body. That was something I'd never heard before. You don't normally realize what's going on in there.' These technologically mediated sounds offered patients a way to hear inside themselves, or rather, stimulated them to imagine what was taking place inside their own bodies.

The other auto-auscultation

Medical vocabulary makes a distinction between 'signs' and 'symptoms'. Definitions for each vary, but here I use 'symptoms' to refer to the patient's experience of a particular problem and 'signs' to refer to indications of disease which may be detected by the patient but which also make a disease apparent to others, particularly those trained to recognize or elicit evidence of illness. Heart sounds and particularly heart murmurs tend to be positioned as signs that guide the clinical understanding of underlying heart problems. Below, however, I describe instances of auto-auscultation in which abnormally loud heart murmurs are heard. Although recognized straight away as abnormal and as a clear cause for concern as a sign of underlying ill-health, these unusually loud sounds may also be understood as symptoms (or at least, they complicate a sign/symptom distinction) because they become a primary means through which patients actually recognize and experience themselves as ill.

A doctor named Harold Segall describes instances of 'auto-auscultation', in which a person actually hears sounds emanating from his or her own body in a letter to the editor of the *American Heart Journal* (1976:269). Segall cites a case study by William Osler who in 1880 published his observations on 'a remarkable heart murmur heard at a distance from the chest wall' (Osler 1880, cited Segall 1976:269). The patient was a twelve year old girl, referred to Osler by one Dr Buller who 'had noticed a remarkable whistling sound while examining her eyes' (ibid.). On auscultation the murmur could not be heard while the child was sitting up in a chair. When she stood, however, Osler observed that 'a loud systolic murmur is heard at the apex, high-pitched, somewhat musical, of maximum intensity in [the] fifth interspace; it varies a good deal, being loud for three or four beats, and then faint for one or two succeeding ones, due to the influence of respiration. On removal of the ear from the chest wall, the murmur can be heard at a distance of several inches' (ibid.). Osler noted that on asking the girl to lean forward and relax the chest 'the murmur was heard with greatly increased intensity. It was distinctly audible at a distance of three feet two inches by measurement, and could be heard at any point on the chest and on top of the head' (ibid.).

Segall goes on to introduce his own case study of a young woman of twenty-three. She also first heard a noise emanating from her chest when she was twelve years old. Segall writes: '[s]he remembers that one day when at home, seated in the company of several friends, she became aware of a particular "squeaking, grating noise", a rhythmically recurring noise emanating from her chest' (ibid.:272). This type of sound is sometimes known as a 'whoop', because of its similarity to the whoop of whooping cough, or a 'honk', because of its likeness to the honk of wild geese (Pickering 1972:731). Though she heard the noise at times over the next ten years she did not consult a doctor until she was eighteen, when she complained of irregularities in her heartbeat. The doctor she saw reassured her, but over the following years the noise began to reappear with increasing frequency until it became noticeable several times a day, at which point she sought further medical advice. Segall continues: '[i]n search of some correlation with a particular activity, she has noticed that it tends to come on when she is standing in the kitchen and vigorously stirring a mixture of food she is preparing. Emotional excitement also tends to elicit the noise' (1976:272). Segall notes that eighty-five years separate Osler's case from his own, but speculates that the two cases had the same or similar underlying physiology, 'a mid-systolic buckling of the mitral valve' (ibid.).

Osler's case study also acts as the background to an article by Fiddler and Scott (1980) entitled 'Heart murmurs audible across the room in children with mitral valve prolapse'. These doctors give case studies of three patients in whom unusually loud heart murmurs have been detected. In the first, a ten year old girl is described as having 'a one-year history of an intermittent sound emanating from her chest in time with the heartbeat. The sound was never present when she visited her family doctor, but was loud enough to be tape recorded at home by her parents...The recording revealed a high pitched "whooping sound"' (ibid.:201). In the second case, a girl once again of twelve years of age had 'noticed an intermittent noise from her chest during the previous three months and on several occasions it had been heard by her parents in the same room' (ibid.:202). The third case was a boy of ten who had previously been admitted to hospital with pericarditis, and 'while straining to vomit, suddenly became aware of a squeaking noise coming from his chest. The noise was also heard by his parents on entering his bedroom and caused them great concern' (ibid.).

Fiddler and Scott point out that several reviews mention patients who are aware of their own murmurs, though only seven, including Osler's famous case, have ever been described in detail (ibid.:202–3). However, as the title of their article indicates, they are confident that these extraordinary murmurs can be attributed to mitral valve prolapse. This condition is thought to occur when one or both leaflets of the mitral valve (there are two in a normal heart), instead of closing cleanly together as the left atrium pumps blood into the left ventricle, billow back into the atrium. The murmur is created by the rush of blood through this prolapsed valve under the strong 'pumping' pressure of the ventricle in systole.

The cases of extreme auto-auscultation described above are interesting because they are so unusual. In general the body contains the heart sounds in such a way that they are certainly inaudible to others, and only distantly audible to the owner of the body him or herself. When these sounds become loud to a person and even the people around him or her, the experience might well be an embarrassing and frightening one. In these instances the volume of the murmurs renders the individual boundaries of the body permeable. The sounds of the heart protrude; as we saw with electrocardiography and echocardiography in Chapter 2, the inside of the body projects into the world in strange auditory forms (Benthien 2002:38).

During my fieldwork I did not meet any patients with murmurs so loud that they could be heard across a room. One patient I saw in Dr Coltart's outpatient clinic had a very loud murmur known as a 'shunt' caused by blood rushing through a small hole in the septum (the muscular wall separating the vessels of the left side of the heart from those of the right). A roaring sound could be heard with the naked ear up to about six inches from the chest. I did, however, meet several patients who had had the experience of being able to hear their own heart sounds, usually because of a serious underlying disorder. In one case a particular auto-acoustic experience caused a frightening distortion of normality.

The patient in question had been admitted to the hospital with terrible headaches, joint stiffness and pouring sweats. I was introduced to him by one of the teaching doctors because his pulse was medically interesting. His was a collapsing pulse. With a normal pulse in the wrist, although there is a tangible build-subside, there remains a degree of constant pressure in the blood vessels of the arm. With a collapsing pulse, however, the fluctuation is far more severe. It feels almost as if the blood is rushing up, and then being quickly sucked back down the arm with each pulse. Holding a thumb across the inside of the patient's elbow and lifting the arm it is possible to feel the blood knock against the thumb as it falls back down the blood vessels. The collapsing pulse is also known as a 'water hammer pulse' or 'Corrigan's sign'. It leads to the expectation of an early diastolic murmur in the aortic area as the aortic valve is not closing properly and the blood, when pumped up the arm, is not kept at pressure by the closing valve. Instead it flows back into the ventricle through the valve, creating turbulence in the blood that produces a murmur.

This patient turned out to be friendly and happy to talk. He described how one night as his illness was just beginning and his temperature was running high, he had been lying on his bed at home and heard a strange rasping noise. The room was dark and he could see nothing, so he chose to ignore the sound at first. When he lay down again, however, he heard the sound a second time. He still could not think what the sound was but assumed that a cat must have got into the room through an open window. When he got up he could find no sign of a cat. Suspicious of his sanity because of his high fever, he tried to sleep once more but soon heard the sound again. This time he got up quickly, convinced there must be a burglar in his flat. A former boxer, he moved around the room throwing punches into the darkness. But having thoroughly searched and found nothing, he lay down once again. This time, as he rested his head on his arm, he realized that the noise was coming from the raging flow of blood inside his body.

Another patient who could hear his own heart sounds had recently been diagnosed with pancreatic cancer. It was very upsetting to see him, as he appeared to my untrained eye to be in good health. He was sitting up in bed and generally spoke in a lively manner, but had been told just two days before not to expect to live more than another three years. He was being kept in hospital for an operation on his pancreas that was expected to take place in the next two days. However, he also had a severe heart murmur. He was able to hear it squeaking whenever he rested his head against the pillow. He remarked, with great sadness in his voice, that it sounded 'like his life draining away'. This would seem to be an example of listening to the body, not just as Henriques says 'symptomatically, as with a doctor's stethoscope to the chest', but 'sympathetically with... hearts open to its song' (2003:472).

Several patients in the cardiothoracic wards also reported being able to hear their own heart murmurs, particularly those people who had loud ejection systolic murmurs that can produce quite a strident squeaking sound. Murmurs tended to be particularly audible to patients when they were lying down and the ward was at its quietest, for instance late at night. In these cases, although the sounds had been made subject to professional medical scrutiny and allocated particular clinical significance, they were also a prominent aspect of the patients' immediate experience of themselves as sick bodies.

Heart sounds, hexis and dys-appearance

In Chapter 5 I introduced Bourdieu's concept of 'hexis', which refers to a set of socially conditioned habits that have become second nature. The term is a shorthand for describing a state of being which encompasses 'a lasting, generalised relation to one's own body, a way of bearing one's body, presenting it to others, moving it, making space for it...' (Bourdieu 1986:474). It is 'a durable manner of standing, speaking, and thereby *feeling* and *thinking* (Bourdieu 1977:93–4, original italics). Hexis, then, as well as referencing physical comportment and bearing, also includes qualities or characteristics in the perception and experience of oneself and one's own body.

Writing on the ultrasound scan, Draper (2002) explores the manner in which this technology has shifted the dynamics of the pregnancy experience. She draws on Duden's concept of 'hexis' which has a slightly different though related emphasis to that of Bourdieu (ibid.:781). Duden uses hexis to refer to 'the habitual state in which a person finds him or herself' (Duden 1993:91). Draper suggests that prior to the rise of foetal ultrasound a woman's pregnancy hexis was characterized by 'hapsis', which she describes as 'knowledge accumulated about the world and experience through perception and touch' (2002:781). She continues: '[a] haptic hexis, therefore, was woman's embodied experience of her pregnancy gained through touch, feeling and being' (ibid.). Draper argues that when foetal ultrasound was introduced the fundamental axis of the pregnancy experience shifted from one based on a haptic hexis to one organized around engagement with a visual image.

The point I wish to make through Draper is that the soundscape of the body is also interlinked with a haptic hexis. Body sounds are strongly connected to notions of touch, feeling and being as much as purely acoustic experience. To use an obvious example, a person running fast may be conscious of the sound of his or her heart beating. However, that person will also experience the heart pounding in his or her chest, feel the sensation of blood pumping in his or her ears, have a sense of being invigorated or perhaps tired. Acoustic, tactile and affective experiences merge. In a similar way, a person may distinctly hear his or her stomach gurgling but at the same time will be aware of vibrations rippling through his or her gut and may, for instance, feel hungry or pleasantly full. The body sounds are intertwined in this wider body hexis.

Normally, the body is experienced as quiet. Its sounds are only at the fringes of our consciousness. As Ackerman points out, 'we rarely hear the internal workings of our body, the caustic churning of our stomach, the whooshing of our blood, the flexing of our joints, our eyelids' relentless opening and closing' (1990:178). It was suggested above that a body in 'sound health', like the ideal modern city, is quietly rhythmical. It contains its internal sounds, which scarcely intrude upon consciousness. In the somewhat disturbing examples of auto-auscultation given above, however, heart sounds become exaggerated and disproportionate. They receive a definite emphasis in the complex sensory and affective interplay within and through which bodies are experienced. The sounds become part of what Leder calls a bodily 'dys-appearance', an unwanted consciousness of the body or aspect of the body that occurs during times of disease, distress or dysfunction (1990:69).

Sound health

When listening to their own bodies as part of their training, the medical students tended to practice auto-auscultation in brief if concentrated spells. Their increased attention to their own heart sounds was not usually long-lasting. In the vast majority of cases they found healthy heart sounds and could draw on what they heard as an index of their sound health. Auto-auscultation did, though, generally have the effect of drawing attention to or amplifying the sonic aspect of the body hexis. Also, for any students who did not immediately hear what they took to be normal sounds, auto-auscultation could produce or exacerbate anxieties over what constitutes a healthy body and how a healthy body should sound.

Rousseau (2003) posits two distinct spheres of thought that come into play in relation to disease. There is a medicalized disorder, framed in medical terminology, and an imagined disorder that is generally held in the consciousness of the person diagnosed. The 'medicalized' and 'imagined' disorder, however, can become intertwined or elided as medical interpretations are integrated into a person's understanding of his or her condition. Medical and anatomical knowledge influence and inform the subjective experience of the body, its workings and processes.

The Turkish man to whom I spoke, for instance, had from quite an early stage understood the clinical significance of his murmur. Hearing it became part of the medical explanation offered by his doctor friend, and the murmur itself became assimilated into his (already medicalized) understanding and experience of his condition. This was also true for the patient introduced in the previous chapter who was invited to listen to the murmur associated with her aortic aneurism. Those patients who were able to hear abnormal sounds issuing from inside themselves without the stethoscope (thereby suffering a particularly acute and disturbing form of auto-auscultation) could find themselves engaged, initially at least, in an unmediated, direct and dramatic sonically-marked experience of the diseased body-as-self. These experiences were, however, quickly informed and shaped by clinical explanations as to the origin and significance of the sounds in question.

In Chapter 2 I introduced Mol's (2002) notion that by applying their respective specialist methods and technologies, medical professionals in hospitals produce related but nonetheless distinctly different 'versions' of the diseased body. Lay ways of 'doing' the body also become evident in the hospital as patients enact their particular 'versions' of their bodies through their experience of illness symptoms and through perceiving the impact of diseases on their lives (ibid.:84). Mol suggests that these medical and lay versions of the body 'hang together', so that we do not encounter a single, unified body in hospitals, but rather many 'variants' of the body (ibid.:115). In the same chapter I argued that sounds become involved in the production of particular versions of heart disease. Tones or noises generated by technologies such as the electrocardiogram and echocardiogram may guide interpretations made by medical professionals as to the health of hearts. When overheard by patients (who are likely not to be medically trained) these sounds may also become involved in 'lay ways' of 'doing' heart disease (ibid.:27, 20). Distinctive sonic versions of the body become audible.

The material introduced in this book so far might broadly be understood to indicate that the listening practices of doctors and other medical professionals are directed towards the body and characterized by diagnostic objectivity, while those of patients are directed towards sounds in the environment and are more subjective and imaginative in nature. In fact, though, examining auto-auscultation as practised by medical students and patients we see some striking similarities of perspective. Auto-auscultation is a type of listening that allows both medical students and patients to engage with the sounds of their own hearts. People in both groups recognize that hearing and understanding the heart sounds can be difficult, and that the listening experience may be fraught with anxiety. They each engage in an objectification of heart sounds, but also interpret them in imaginative ways. Distinctions between professional and lay versions of the audible body, then, are by no means stark or clearly drawn here; frames of reference and experience converge. In auto-auscultation it is arguably the singularity, rather than the multiplicity of the heard body that is striking.

But while in the instances of auto-auscultation described above the orientation of medical students and patients to the heart sounds may be similar in broad terms, it is clear that their interpretations and experiences do not exactly correspond. Medical students bring a certain level of diagnostic sophistication to their interpretations of the heart sounds, while patients tend to glean and assemble interpretations from the more or less complete fragments of medical knowledge imparted to them by doctors. The fact that they already understand themselves to be ill also means that, for many patients, the experience of hearing their own heart sounds carries a seriousness and depth unfamiliar to the vast majority of medical students. So while the body as encountered through auto-auscultation cannot be described as multiple, it would evidently not be accurate either to conceptualize it as perfectly unified. Neither quite multiple nor singular, the 'sonorous, sonorized body' is a body whose versions are imperfectly merged, inconsistently overlapping and somewhat messily entangled (Nancy 2007:43).

CHAPTER 8

Deathoscope

Auscultation, Echocardiography and the 'Death of the Stethoscope'

Medical practice is not static. It is in a constant state of change as clinical goals and policies alter, as new technologies are introduced and as the demand for particular skills increases or decreases. This chapter explores a shift that many considered to be occurring within medical practice at the time of my fieldwork. Auscultation as a mode of diagnosis was, some felt, being challenged, undermined or even made obsolete by the increasing use of cardiac ultrasound or echocardiography. Questions were raised as to whether listening skills were in decline and might, in the relatively near future, be rendered unnecessary.

The chapter begins by describing the way in which decisions as to the nature of heart sounds, and specifically of heart murmurs, were negotiated in the clinics I observed at St Thomas'. As was indicated in Chapter 5, the establishment of consensus about what has been heard during auscultation can be challenging, particularly when those sounds are subtle. I examine how seniority and authority within the professional hierarchy of the hospital are mobilized in the discussion and consolidation of findings obtained using auscultation. The chapter goes on to consider the manner in which echocardiography brings about a reconfiguration of the 'network' of human and technological actors involved in the investigation of heart murmurs, at the same time causing a redistribution of authority (Latour 1999:204). Diagnostic power effectively drains away from auscultation and expert auscultators towards echocardiography and those familiar with that technology.

In their work on cochlear inplant debates, Valente *et al.* employ the term 'sensory politics', which they suggest refers to 'the intersection of biological perception and cultural mediation and interpretation within a field of power'

(2011:246). Seeking to reveal the sensory politics underpinning what they view as the promotion of cochlear implants by the 'medical-educational-industrial complex', they argue that the advancement of this type of surgery, in part at least, represents the (not necessarily conscious or intentional) imposition of the sensory dispositions of a hearing majority culture onto a deaf minority culture (ibid.). The concept of sensory politics is useful, they suggest, because it clarifies that arguments in favour of implantation, even those supposedly based on a purely scientific rationale, are in fact filtered through a set of cultural assumptions which express a specific valuation of the senses and of particular perceptual abilities.

This chapter examines what might be described as the 'sensory politics' underpinning the perceived movement of diagnostic authority away from auscultation and towards echocardiography. It does not argue that this change is the consequence of a strategic manipulation effected by one group of medical professionals over another, but rather assesses the different sensory characteristics of stethoscopic listening and echocardiography, examining the different valuations given to visual and auditory 'evidence' in Western medical culture. The chapter identifies a strong preoccupation with visual gazing as the basis of diagnostic knowledge within medicine, driving the enthusiasm for echocardiography as an essentially visual technology.

Speculation over the future of auscultation forms a discourse around the 'death of the stethoscope'. Introducing this discourse, the chapter suggests that it does not simply comprise a debate as to whether or not cardiac ultrasound is 'taking over' from auscultation. Instead, it provides a forum for the articulation of wider anxieties within the medical profession over an increasing use of and dependence upon technology. There is concern that 'technology-creep' may be responsible for a decrease in diagnostic acuity among doctors (Kirsch 1998). The interpersonal skills necessary for the proper practice of 'bedside medicine' are also considered by some to be at risk, as technologies introduce distance and lessen contact between doctors and their patients. These feelings of unease are linked in turn to predictions of deskilling among doctors, and a concurrent devaluation of medical professionals in general. Interestingly, the fact that auscultation requires the acquisition of practical skill and also involves close personal interaction with patients has allowed the instrument to stand for a way of working in which the doctor remains personally resourceful and independent, while sensitive to and understanding of the needs of patients. It is a practice in which the doctor him or herself remains the nexus of medical agency as opposed to being what might be regarded as an essentially administrative link in a series of medically orientated technological processes. In the discourse of the death of the stethoscope, the stethoscope itself has been appropriated as a symbol of what is evidently, for some, a cherished ideal of medical practice.

The chapter concludes by taking up the notion of sensory politics again, examining the appropriation of the stethoscope as an emblem of sympathetic and empathetic medical practice. It refers back to Sterne's (2003a) 'audiovisual litany', a set of repeatedly voiced assumptions about the fundamental nature of hearing and sight. Although, as explored in Chapter 6, in particular contexts the sense of hearing may be linked to the establishment of objective distance or detachment, or to the production of forms of objectification, in Sterne's litany hearing is strongly associated with affective engagement. I suggest that it is this association that allows the stethoscope as an acoustic instrument, and auscultation as an acoustic technique, to reference the compassionate application of clinical skill and to carry its particular symbolic burden in the discourse of the death of the stethoscope. Interestingly, then, sensory politics – perceptions of perception, so to speak – are shown to be at the heart of discussions over the outlook for auscultation. However, at least two different threads of sensory politics are in play. Some argue that stethoscopic listening has low value because as it is not considered (relative to echocardiography for instance) to be a particularly powerful or objective diagnostic technique. At the same time, others suggest that auscultation has high value partly because it can be considered productive of compassionate medical attitudes and interactions. These positions, of course, are not necessarily mutually exclusive, but show that sensory politics can underpin the formation of both pragmatic and moral arguments in discussions over the future of medical practice and the direction that it should take.

Defensive medicine

During fieldwork I was told about a clinic run by a man named Major General James Alex Jonse, a military doctor one of whose responsibilities was to determine whether or not the heart problems detected at military medicals were sufficiently serious to render recently enlisted cadets unfit for training. I was told there would be 'murmurs galore' at his clinic, and that the Major General was known to be an expert auscultator. I obtained permission to attend the clinic, and on the day I visited the Major General came to meet me at reception. Though as I later learned, seventy years old, he was an intimidating man, broad and strong with a firm handshake. He seemed to look down at me even though I was easily taller. His eyes had the look of one well used to scanning inferiors.

'One feels that most young doctors are incompetent auscultators,' he said when we had sat down in his consultation room. 'They don't do it properly. In fact, the medical profession in general is not good at auscultation. Most students are not taught to auscultate properly.' He explained that as a medical student and doctor in Edinburgh he had 'cut [his] teeth on congenital and rheumatic heart disease'. Congenital heart disease refers to problems in the heart that are present from birth. Rheumatic heart disease is caused by rheumatic fever, which can cause damage to the heart valves, meaning that they become stiff and/or misshapen. The flow of blood through these misshapen valves often creates heart murmurs. Rheumatic heart disease is still seen in Britain, though it is rare. However, the Major General told me that when he began to practise medicine in the early sixties, auscultation was effectively *the* major technique for the diagnosis of these types of heart disease. Indeed, he described auscultation as being 'more or less on its own, and as a consequence taken extremely seriously' in both teaching and practice. For the Major General a clear generational divide was evident in the diagnostic skills of doctors his age and those of younger doctors and, in particular, medical students.

After giving his views on the current state of auscultation, the Major General explained that military personnel undergo arduous training which involves putting a great deal of stress on the heart. A thorough investigation of any suspected heart problems is therefore essential in order to ensure not only that new recruits are sufficiently healthy to endure their training, but also that the Ministry of Defence (MoD) has protected itself against potential legal claims from cadets and their families in the event of death or injury linked to heart disease. Appropriately for a clinic run by the MoD, this is known as 'defensive medicine'.

There was a knock at the door, and the doctor opened it. A nervous boy/man entered the room and took a seat next to the Major General's desk. The Major General spoke to me as though the cadet were not there. 'This is fairly typical of what we get in here', he said, passing over a piece of paper. It was a referral letter from the doctor who had given the cadet his introductory medical. He had detected a soft, grade II ejection-systolic murmur at the cadet's left sternal edge and wanted it to be investigated further. The Major General took a brief history from the lad as I read the letter, asking him his age, how he occupied his time, was he a drinker or a smoker and so on. Then he told him to take off his top things and lie on the couch.

The Major General's tone and actions were brisk and efficient. Voicing concern once again that medical students today are not taught auscultation properly, he explained each stage of the examination as he performed it. To begin with, he said, one should inspect the hands and skin, then feel each of the femoral arteries (which are found at the inner thigh where the tape measure is held if an inside leg measurement is being taken) while taking the pulse to check that the blood is circulating evenly around the body. Next one should observe the veins in the neck and palpate the chest for 'heaves' and 'thrills', which are vibrations in the heart, sometimes referred to as 'palpable murmurs'. Then one should feel the pulse in the wrist and auscultate the heart and the carotid artery in the neck. Asking the boy to sit up and take deep breaths, the Major General then listened at three points down his spine, during which, he said, he was listening for sounds from the lungs that might indicate asthma or breathing problems. Finally, asking his patient to lie over on his left side, the Major General listened again to the mitral area of the heart with the bell of his stethoscope. He then gestured to me. I put on my stethoscope and approached the cadet to do the same examination. Each doctor has his own particular style of performing auscultation. The Major General's was characterized by a rigour and physicality I had not seen before but imagined was typical of military doctors. I tried to conduct the examination in exactly the same way as he had done.

When I had finished the Major General told the boy to 'dress up' and to go upstairs for an echocardiogram. As indicated in Chapter 2, echocardiography can produce detailed real-time images of the heart as it beats. These images can show, for instance, the working of the heart valves and the extent and direction of blood flow across those valves. The technology also allows measurements to be taken of the thickness of the heart muscle at chosen points. If a cardiac abnormality is found in a patient in the UK it is increasingly standard practice for that patient to be sent for an echocardiogram. Just as foetal ultrasound has become part of the 'normal pregnancy package', echocardiography has become part of routine cardiac investigation (Draper 2002:778).

In the diagnosis and investigation of heart murmurs at his clinic, then, the Major General would assess the opinion of the military doctor, who in some cases was in turn assessing the opinion of a General Practitioner. But even if a murmur was identified and confirmed by both or all three doctors, what the Major General described as 'paper proof' was still required before its existence and severity could be certified beyond doubt. It was as if the murmur initially floated free, unsubstantiated, a little cloud of uncertainty, becoming more fixed and solid as one doctor confirmed the opinion of another. The murmur's existence was only certified beyond any doubt after a review of the findings obtained through echocardiography. In the case of the cadet described above, the Major General explained that there was a slight murmur present, and so he could not describe the heart as clinically normal. However, he suspected that the echocardiogram would show it to be 'normal enough' for the Major General to pass him as fit. When, twenty minutes later, the results of the scan came back, the two words printed at the top of the paper did indeed read 'Normal Scan'. The detail reported normal functioning on each valve except for 'trivial tricuspid regurgitation' that, as the Major General had indicated, was not sufficiently serious to warrant keeping the cadet out of active service. The military doctor, the Major General and the echocardiogram were in accord.

Authority and the echocardiogram

The Major General's clinic illustrates that a murmur becomes objectively present partly through a consensus of diagnostic opinion between doctors. There is a sense that objectivity is 'the achievement of inter-subjective confirmation and acceptance' (Moran 2000:61). As described in Chapter 5, however, establishing an inter-subjective consensus on findings made through auscultation can be difficult. The perceptual isolation of individual listeners and the complexity of articulating the particularities of heard sounds mean that although objectivity born of 'inter-subjective confirmation' might be relatively easy to establish with simple heart sounds, it is notoriously difficult where more subtle sounds are concerned.

Examining what he describes as the social construction of scientific facts, Latour (1987) considers the authorship of scientific articles. He notes that this kind of text is made 'for attack or defence' (ibid.:61). One important strategy of defence, Latour explains, is to build up a body of support through connecting one's argument to those of other people. If someone wishes to refute the position one adopts in an article, he or she will then have to go back and also refute the findings of all those whose work has been incorporated into it (ibid.:44). For Latour, the more a piece of scientific literature draws on the work of others, the more 'social' and hence the stronger it is (ibid.:62). The same is true of academic writing. Authors quote the work of others in order to reinforce their arguments; indeed, I do so (using Latour) in this very paragraph, an irony that would not be lost on Latour himself. But in a similar way, within the hospital doctors attempt to consolidate their diagnoses partly through gaining confirmation from other doctors. Approval by a colleague gives weight to findings and makes them firmer. In drawing on the support of colleagues, then, doctors produce social diagnoses, and, in cases like that described above, social murmurs.

Of the actors who might be involved in the production of a social text or diagnosis, some will of course carry more authority than others. Within the hospital, the authority that a doctor commands is, broadly speaking, linked to his or her position in the professional hierarchy. This hierarchy is in turn an index of his or her relative level of knowledge, experience and skill. One junior doctor I spoke to explained to me that, in his team, while Senior House Officers and registrars might carry out examinations on patients and discover murmurs, those murmurs were only speculative diagnoses until the consultant had listened and decided that he agreed with the finding. Sometimes senior doctors such as Dr Coltart would disagree with the findings made by more junior doctors. Their seniority meant that it was their evaluation of the murmur that was carried forward. They commanded the authority to dictate what had been heard.

In one of the cases I observed at the Major General's clinic, he was sceptical as to the presence of a murmur that a military doctor claimed to have identified in a cadet. When my turn came to listen I thought I could hear a soft murmur, a kind of thickening of the first heart sound, but the Major General was unconvinced and shook his head. He reiterated his opinion that there was no murmur and stated that if there was one it was so trifling as to be insignificant. The echocardiogram, he said, would indicate a normal scan. When the results came back a normal report was indeed given. As the most senior doctor involved, the Major General's opinion would have prevailed over that of the first military doctor. Ultimately, though, he validated his diagnosis through the findings of the echocardiogram. It was the person carrying out the echocardiogram and interpreting the data who had given the definitive assessment of the condition of the patient's heart valves.

In a similar way, on one occasion during fieldwork, Rishi and I went to see a patient in the St Thomas' Hospital Lupus Unit. One of the latest developments in her condition had been the discovery of a heart murmur which had been detected by one of the doctors charged with her care, a microbiology specialist. This doctor had said it was a soft, pan-systolic murmur and added that he believed the lady to have contracted endocarditis (a bacterial infection of the heart) that was now affecting one of her valves. Another more senior doctor had then listened and described the murmur as 'only *very* soft.' He had referred the patient for a TOE (trans-oesophageal echocardiogram), a procedure in which a small ultrasound transducer is passed down the throat, often allowing particularly detailed images of the valves to be produced as the ultrasound waves are not attenuated by body fat or bone as can be the case when the transducer is moved across the surface of the chest. The senior doctor who had conducted the TOE, however, said there was no indication of any stenosis or regurgitation. He felt the valves were normal.

The patient told us that she herself had been suspicious of the microbiologist's diagnosis. She said she felt he was 'using' the murmur, 'hearing things' as she put it, in order to secure control over her treatment. She said she knew the two senior doctors to be experts in their fields and felt that the other doctor was 'comparatively young, inexperienced and self-interested.' She implied that what is heard depends on who is listening. The first doctor, she believed, was influenced by his desire to take control of her treatment through his own particular medical specialization, as hearing a murmur and diagnosing endocarditis would strengthen the case for her to be treated as a microbiology patient. But this doctor's 'inclination of the ear', so to speak, might not be shared by a doctor with a different specialism or one with no vested interest in a particular diagnostic outcome.

In this instance, the first doctor was obliged to offer his opinion on what he had heard to a second, more senior doctor. The first doctor half agrees and half disagrees with what the first doctor says he has found. The murmur is 'only *very* soft'. It is almost as if he is trying to give the opinion that there is no murmur without offending the first doctor. On the basis of auscultation, then, the murmur has only a flimsy half-existence through the half-consensus of these two doctors. Ultimately, though, the patient is sent for an echocardiogram and it is these findings that are taken as the definitive statement on whether or not blood is leaking across the valve. The echocardiogram shows that the valve is functioning normally, and so the murmur effectively evaporates. Once again, the evidence of the echocardiogram and the opinion of the doctor who interprets it are given overall authority.

Senses of authority

Why should it be that findings produced by echocardiography are endowed with more authority than those generated through auscultation? There are several points to cover in answering this question. The most obvious concerns the nature of the echocardiogram, which, as indicated above, produces 'a graphic and quantitative depiction of body events', creating detailed images of the heart and its workings, allowing for a close assessment of the level and direction of blood flow across the heart valves and permitting measurements of layers of the heart muscle (Reiser 1993:264). The technology generates information that simply cannot be obtained through an examination of the heart made by the doctor using a stethoscope or by recourse to his senses alone. Echocardiography, when properly performed, provides greater diagnostic detail than auscultation.

As discussed in Chapter 3, the adoption of the stethoscope in nineteenth century medical practice represented part of a more general shift away from doctors depending solely on the illness narratives of patients towards growing independence based on the capacity of medical men to make observations through the application of their own, trained senses. Doctors were increasingly able to base their diagnoses on what were perceived to be objective assessments rather than depending on the subjective accounts of illness experiences given by their patients. But Reiser suggests that in the later nineteenth and early twentieth century, doctors became increasingly aware of the fact that empirical observation was itself not immune to bias: '[w]ho knew what the doctor heard, saw or felt; or how the events of the previous day, the nature of previous medical training, or even the mark of heredity influenced the perception?' (ibid.:266). There was recognition that the sensory impulses experienced by the doctor could not be referenced to any meaningfully independent or standardized measure. Uncertainty over the precise nature of the sensory signal perceived by the doctor also meant it was impossible to verify that a particular signal had been appropriately interpreted. As they were introduced, technologies such as the thermometer, X-ray and electrocardiogram – which independently registered numerical, pictorial and graphic evidence – later came to be considered superior to the doctor's senses because they were perceived to be more objective (ibid.:267).

Reiser also points out that the above technologies offered additional benefits in terms of communication. The codification and comparison of heard signs in the body is problematic for those practising auscultation today just as it was for the pioneers of the practice. The difficulty of couching sensory experience in language is also apparent when considering evidence gathered through the other senses, for example the sense of touch when feeling the pulse (ibid.:268). However, technologies such as X-ray, electrocardiography and importantly for the current discussion, ultrasound, offer numerical, graphical and pictorial data that are amenable to simultaneous viewing by doctors, their colleagues and students. Medical professionals are immediately provided with shared reference points that readily allow discussion and comparison. These advantages also mean that information obtained through echocardiography is likely to be assigned more credibility and value in terms of objectivity than assessments made drawing on the senses of the physician alone.

Of course, echocardiography also relies on the senses of the person who operates the technology and interprets the data it produces. The sonographer must co-ordinate his or her sight, touch and to some extent, hearing when moving the transducer over the chest. He or she must make selections as to where and how the transducer is directed. At the same time, the assessment of the data produced during an echocardiogram is essentially a hermeneutic or interpretive practice. Diagnoses are not absolute but can be challenged and revised. Echocardiography might, then, seem to be as prone to subjective bias as any technique involving more direct application of the doctor's senses to the patient's body. However, the fact that echocardiography ultimately produces visible and legible data allows a transparency in relation to diagnostic findings and decision-making that is not permitted by what might be regarded as more immediate sensory techniques.

Comparing echocardiography and auscultation, then, it might be argued that echocardiographic findings have more authority than those produced through auscultation because visual evidence is 'naturally' more substantial or concrete than the evidence provided by sounds. Sounds are fleeting, transient and insubstantial (at least in a time and place where recording is not available). Othello's request that Iago show him the 'ocular', rather than the auricular proof of Desdemona's infidelity, for instance, seems to be common sense (Act III, scene iii, line 366). But the weight attributed to visual and auditory evidence respectively is subject to cultural variation. Gell, for instance, describes how among the Umeda of Papua New Guinea it is sounds that are favoured as proof in what he describes as 'conflicts over evidence' (1995:238). Audible but invisible or concealed objects are considered to be 'present' in a way that is difficult for Westerners to grasp. Thus, for instance, when one man describes to a sceptical Gell how he came across an ogre on a forest path, it is the sound rather than the appearance of the ogre to which he makes repeated reference in asserting the truth of the encounter. Within European society, however, as Bloch (2008) argues, there is a historically well-established connection between seeing and truth. He points out that the English word 'evidence' is based on the Latin verb *videre*: to see (ibid.:22). Though admitting the existence of exceptions, Bloch suggests that there is a general association between truth and sight among peoples across the world, with a correspondingly high value placed on visual evidence.

The strong link between seeing and knowing in Western culture, through which visual evidence becomes highly valued in the establishment of truth, has also been noted in work on the history of science, and importantly, of medicine (Jenks 1995). Thus, Foucault (1973) argues that, during medicine's anatomical turn, the patient body came to be positioned as an object consisting of internal and external layers and surfaces to be opened up and made visible to the eyes of medical men through autopsy (ibid.:8). It was the evidence provided by what was seen that came to be fundamental to the production of evidence-based medical knowledge. Draper observes that 'in the 21st century the medical gaze is no longer dependent on the corpse for its mapping of the human body' (2002:777). She points to the new technological dissection of the living body made possible by, for instance, Computerized Axial Tomography (or CAT scanning), Magnetic Resonance Imaging (MRI) and, importantly, ultrasound. These technologies, she suggests, embody a preoccupation with looking and the use of visual evidence in the production of knowledge that pervades Western medicine.

Foucault recognizes that the concept of the medical gaze encompasses more than is suggested by the word 'gaze' alone, and should be regarded as 'pluri-sensorial' (1973:165). He notes the importance of listening and touching in the production of medical knowledge, and even envisages Laennec listening to a patient's chest (ibid.). But Foucault maintains that in listening with his stethoscope, Laennec is still haunted by a visual diagnostic image that he is attempting to realize through sound (ibid.). For Foucault there is in the end 'an absolute, absolutely integrating gaze' that dominates and structures medical perception (ibid.:167). In echocardiography, a process of conversion or transcription takes place in which the technology creates actual, rather than, as Foucault suggests is the case with auscultation, anticipated or imagined visual images. The body is made accessible to the eye, rather than the mind's eye. Sonography means 'drawing in sound' and this is what takes place. It is clear, then, that cardiac ultrasound belongs more immediately to what Duden calls medicine's 'visual command performance' than auscultation (1993:21). Echocardiography's capacity to realise and fulfil rather than anticipate a visual medical gaze partly explains why it was considered by many to hold more authority than auscultation as a diagnostic technique at the time of my fieldwork.

To return to a consideration of the sensory politics underpinning an investment of diagnostic authority in echocardiography over auscultation, it is clear that there is a strong cultural preference for seeing as a route to the production of clinical evidence and diagnostic objectivity within modern medicine. Techniques of listening have played and continue to play an important role in the generation of medical knowledge. They arguably only do so, however, in interplay with vision, and with the aim of producing an acoustic illumination, a visualization of the bodily interior through sound. Diagnostic listening can be understood as subsumed within a deeper cultural and ideological investment in vision within medicine, which is reflected in an overwhelming investment of both resources and authority in visual diagnostics.

The 'death of the stethoscope'

I found during my research that while many medical students recognized the importance of the stethoscope in asserting their status as doctors in waiting, and knew that they would be obliged to acquire some skill in auscultation in order to pass their exams, they were less convinced that once they had qualified auscultation would be of substantial use to them in diagnosis. Stethoscopic listening might be helpful in making an initial assessment of whether or not a patient's heart was normal. Should any abnormality be detected, though, they knew they could and indeed would be expected to send that patient for a cardiac ultrasound scan. While echocardiography had not been available for much of the careers of senior doctors such as Dr Coltart or Major General Alex Jonse, the students I encountered knew that cardiac ultrasound meant they would never have to depend heavily on auscultation. 'Who are the nicest people in a hospital?' a medical student once asked me. 'The ultrasound guys,' came the answer. This joke might be understood to have a subtext. Medical students have good reason to like those working in cardiac ultrasound. They spare them the painstaking task of becoming expert auscultators, easing the pressure on their own diagnostic skills.

It seems that medical students, then, feel auscultation will eventually for them be only a preliminary form of investigation, essentially a type of 'triage'. Triage is a system of sorting. The medical sense of the term originated from the handling of war casualties. The wounded were examined briefly and placed into categories, for instance, those who were injured but could wait for attention, those who needed immediate help and those who were so severely hurt that treatment was futile. Triage allowed for limited medical resources to be allocated with maximum efficiency and to optimum effect. Auscultation, the students seemed to suggest, will in future be used in a similar way to sort healthy hearts from those showing abnormal clinical signs such as murmurs. Fine differentiation of those murmurs will be unnecessary, however, as patients will be examined more closely with cardiac ultrasound.

On a number of occasions I heard doctors remark that the stethoscope was 'a dying technology' or that auscultation was 'a dying art'. Of course, in places where the technology is not widely or routinely available, auscultation may still be of vital importance. Zani, a young doctor from Pakistan who was attending St Thomas' in order to qualify to practise in Britain, pointed out that in countries less economically prosperous and medically well-served than those in the West, echocardiography is too expensive for routine use. As a consequence, skill in auscultation is considered highly important. In the relatively well-resourced and technologically sophisticated cardiology unit at St Thomas', however, there was not the same dependency on auscultation. Some doctors felt the prognosis for the technique did not look good.

In addition to the spoken accounts of doctors I was able to locate references to the death of the stethoscope in written sources. Chiming with Major General James Alex Jonse's comment that 'most young doctors are incompetent auscultators', these articles also voiced a concern that the availability of new technologies (echocardiography in particular) was causing an erosion of listening skills and clinical skills more generally (Mangione and Nieman 1997, Kirsch 1998). In a comment that resonates with the Major General's thoughts, Babu (1999) suggests that today's medical students are not being taught auscultation well. He argues that this is because they are obliged to learn from doctors whose own skills have suffered through a culture of over-investment in diagnostic technology within medicine. It is important to bear in mind, however, that the doctors I reference here are commenting on students at American medical schools. Although concern over deteriorating diagnostic skills among students was evident during fieldwork at St Thomas', this anxiety might well be more pronounced in America where is it generally accepted that there is more of a culture of (over) investment in medical technology than in the UK. As I go on to argue below, however, while the discourse of the 'death of the stethoscope' may reflect concerns about the diagnostic acuity of medical students and some medical professionals, it also warns of the dangers of a decay in other aspects of the work and role of the doctor. More than just listening skill is at stake in the imagined or projected death of the stethoscope.

Technostalgia

Porter identifies a long tradition of the doctor being a practitioner of 'bedside medicine', an idea he traces back into medical antiquity (1997:10). He notes that the ideal of an intimate physician-patient relationship was fostered even in the medieval West (ibid.:9–10). The doctor was and still is imagined to be a man (or more recently a woman) who is involved in close, face-to-face contact with the patient. He or she is directly implicated in the patient's suffering, or at least, as Berger suggests, bears witness to it (1967). Porter points out that much is made of the significance of this personal touch in medicine, the face-to-face relationship even being considered 'essential to the office and alchemy of healing' (1997:628).

The cultivation of a good bedside manner was an implicit element of many of the interactions I witnessed in classes during fieldwork. Students would pick up on the small actions and touches of the teaching doctors: concerned nods, murmurs of empathy and understanding. They later reproduced these details themselves in their own interactions with patients. Auscultation in particular offered opportunities to articulate qualities that might be identified with a good bedside manner. The interaction involves the listener getting physically close to the patient and though the extent of that proximity sometimes created awkwardness and embarrassment for students, it also produced chances to express sensitivity and concern. Importantly, the contact generated by stethoscopic listening also offered an opportunity for students to talk to their patients and learn more about them than their diagnostic signs could reveal. As indicated in Chapter 6, Dr Coltart encouraged students to return to a patient to listen again if they had had problems hearing a particular sonic detail during an examination in class. When they did this, the students were sometimes surprised to find themselves falling into conversations in which they heard a great deal about patients' lives and about the circumstances which had brought them to hospital.

Porter indicates that during the anatomical turn, doctors developed proficiency at clinical diagnosis, pursuing an enthusiasm for scientific medicine. They were aided in this effort by important new technologies such as the stethoscope. But as a result of their scientific approach, doctors were sometimes felt to have lost sight of the fact that patients were social beings as well as sick bodies. Medical technologies were perceived to foster clinical detachment and a disengagement from the patient-as-person. Ironically, then, 'at the very time that medicine was improving, a decline in the physician-patient relationship was taking place' (ibid.:683).

Medical technologies have continued to proliferate within the Western medical setting and concern over their impact has risen correspondingly. Of course, there should be no reason why technologies either inevitably or invariably generate detachment or separation between doctor and patient; yet there appears to be some feeling that they can bring about a neglect of the patient: '[T]echnology threatens important humanistic elements of the doctor-patient relationship. Our embrace of medical technology has taken us too far away from the bedside' (Kirsch 1998). I found this sentiment echoed by a number of doctors during fieldwork, but it was perhaps expressed most directly during a conversation outside an echocardiography meeting on the administration floor. One doctor joked sarcastically that this was as close as he ever got to the bedside these days. The other replied that the closest he ever got was reading the name at the top of the test printout. 'What? Isn't a patient just a collection of numbers and forms?' responded the first.

The stethoscope was initially one of the diagnostic instruments that characterized a wider enthusiasm for scientific medicine and as such should arguably be classed among the technologies considered to have driven or be driving doctors and patients apart. Indeed, we have seen how auscultation could produce feelings of objectification and alienation in patients through the particular physical and perceptual distance between doctor and patient that it creates. Yet, evidently caught up in a kind of 'technostalgia', the instrument has been referred to as the 'umbilical cord of medicine', uniting doctor and patient (Pinch and Reinecker 2009, Gerchufsky 1995). The stethoscope is considered to produce not solely a diagnostic interaction, but also a humane one in which an intimate physician-patient relationship may develop. Dr Coltart once described the stethoscope as a way of 'literally getting to the heart of the patient', playing on the notion that the heart is the seat of emotion and feeling rather than simply a mechanism for circulation. In a similar way, the discourse of the 'death of the stethoscope' situates the instrument as a symbol of a sympathetic, humanistic kind of medical practice that some doctors are anxious should not be lost amid the gains offered by new diagnostic technologies.

Technoscepticism

At the time of my fieldwork doctors were not generally responsible for carrying out echocardiograms. Some did possess the necessary knowledge and skill, and one or two were experts in this area. Most routine cardiac ultrasound investigations, however, were left to technicians. I heard a number of conversations about hand-held ultrasound machines that it was believed would soon become available. These were said to be easy to operate and did not require qualified technicians, allowing doctors to use echocardiography themselves at the bedside. At the time of my fieldwork, however, these devices had yet to be introduced and while some doctors were aware of how to interpret the results of echocardiography, the actual performance of the technique was most often outside their professional domain.

It is easy to see that prior to the proliferation of medical technologies and, particularly for the purposes of this discussion, echocardiography, the 'network' of relationships between people and technologies used in making a diagnosis could be considered relatively simple (Latour 1999:204). Investigating a heart murmur, for example, the doctor would 'enlist' the stethoscope and engage his own skill, knowledge and powers of judgment in examining a patient, often later conferring with other doctors (ibid.:178). Following the introduction of echocardiography, however, that network of diagnostic relationships became widened and extended. New machines, technicians and experts became involved in decision-making. Within this reconfiguration of people and technology an important change takes place: diagnostic agency becomes more widely dispersed and the doctor is no longer necessarily the key locus of medical expertise.

Over the course of my fieldwork I noticed that Dr Coltart told all his students about the time he had spent at Stanford University. He related how at this prestigious medical school he had impressed his colleagues with his bedside diagnostic skills. 'How do you know that?' they would ask him after he had made a diagnosis. 'Have you seen the test results already?' Dr Coltart said he would reply that there was no need as the diagnosis was already plain to him. He felt that there tended to be an over-dependence on test results in American medicine, and suggested that this type of medical culture was increasingly prevalent in Britain. It seemed that Dr Coltart told his students this story as a kind of fable, one which urged them to sharpen and practise their physical diagnosis skills and encouraged them to adopt a kind of medicine which did not entail over-dependency on tests.

Of course, doctors' reliance on a range of technologies and the skills of those who operate them is not new. They have for a long time used, for instance, the results of blood tests, X-rays, cultures and so on in reaching diagnoses. But Dr Coltart's story of his time at Stanford might be interpreted as a kind of polemic, urging new doctors to resist this trend, to safeguard their own skills by using and applying them. In a similar way, the discourse of the death of the stethoscope warns of the loss of important skills that may result from a technophile culture of over-investment of money, training and faith in medical technologies. It expresses a certain technoscepticism and a reluctance to accept that advances in diagnostic technology inevitably represent improvements in medical practice. At the same time, the discourse taps into a wider anxiety among medical professionals around what is known as 'de-skilling'.

Haug (1988) suggests that de-skilling in the medical profession has been a subject of discussion for almost twenty years, the sophistication of computers being perceived as a threat to medical judgment. Rather than being a definite or specific problem, however, Haug indicates that de-skilling is a pervasive but nebulous angst within the medical profession. It should be pointed out that concerns over de-skilling are not linked to advances in diagnostic technology alone. Lupton (1997) suggests that other factors, including threats to the autonomy of physicians created by the state, are also implicated in the issue. Increasing dependence on diagnostic technologies, however, remains a common worry among the doctors in her study.

Of course, the stethoscope is a technology of a kind, but it is a technology that requires a well-practised, actively sensing user, the locus of, among other things, a specialized auditory knowledge. In the discourse of the death of the stethoscope, the stethoscope partly stands for the doctor as the nexus of diagnostic agency. It is adopted as a symbol both of the value of tacit knowledge and a rejection of the notion that all medical expertise can be objectively and technologically rendered. The 'death' of the stethoscope as a result of an increasing dependence on more advanced technologies might have serious consequences. Where the doctor becomes simply a point for the collation of test results, the value of his or her role and that of the entire profession will fall. The doctor will no longer be irreplaceable as a holder and bearer of knowledge and experience. Instead, he or she will become a more ancillary figure in the administration of medical knowledge.

Clinging on

Predictions of the death of the stethoscope are evidently not new. Shindler points out that the instrument's demise has been 'wrongly but repeatedly foretold over the years' (2004:51). He relates the tale of an early twentieth century radiologist who placed a stethoscope on display in a coffin-shaped case. 'It was his mistaken belief that X-ray of the heart would shortly render the stethoscope obsolete' (ibid.). I certainly did not see evidence of stethoscopes being consigned to drawers or dustbins at St Thomas'; indeed, this book as a whole suggests that cardiac auscultation still has considerable importance in the curriculum for medical students, and given that the students with whom I conducted fieldwork would qualify within two years it seems unlikely that they will be the generation of doctors who certify the stethoscope dead. Rather, they give at least some assurance of its ongoing life. These students, however, will not be as dependent on their stethoscopes as previous generations of doctors have been. The aim of this chapter, though, is not to reach a conclusion about the future of auscultation, but to expose some of the sensory politics underpinning the ways in which auscultation has been conceptualized and used to both motivate and resist change within medicine.

Above I described how concerns over the death of the stethoscope articulate anxieties over the devaluation or disappearance of the more humane elements of medical practice. The stethoscope has come to symbolize these elements because it creates a space for intimate conversation, the establishment of rapport, the expression of care and concern and so on. I would suggest, however, that it is not coincidence that an acoustic technology should have been chosen to bear this particular symbolic burden.

In Chapter 6 I introduced Sterne's concept of the 'audiovisual litany', a set of assertions that he observes are repeatedly made about the difference between hearing and vision (2003a:15). I selected the following contrasts from Sterne's more extensive list, using them to argue that auscultation in fact presents instances where hearing produces perceptual effects more often associated with vision:

> Hearing immerses its subject, vision offers a perspective.
> Hearing places us inside an event, seeing gives us a perspective on the event.
> Hearing tends towards subjectivity, vision towards objectivity.
> Hearing is about affect, vision is about intellect.

Taking the last two of these contrasts, it would certainly seem that, in the discourse of the death of the stethoscope, auscultation is attacked or regarded by some as inadequate because of what is considered the inherent subjectivity or compromised objectivity of the technique. Visual technologies such as echocardiography, on the other hand, are considered to enable the achievement of a robust clinical objectivity. At the same time, others argue that technologies including echocardiography produce a perceptual distance and detachment that creates an overly intellectualized engagement with physiology and pathology. Through a kind of technostalgia, they defend auscultation, associating it with interactions that, though not necessarily productive of affective responses, bring doctor and patient close and encourage a certain degree of empathy in exchanges between them. Thus, for example, Kirsch is able to make the assertion that in the act of auscultation, 'a message of caring and concern is communicated' (1998). He also suggests that the stethoscope should serve as a reminder of the importance of listening to patients' accounts of their illnesses: '[p]atients…beseech us to listen to them.

How can we learn to do this better? Perhaps the stethoscopes dangling round our necks or stuffed into our pockets can remind us of this mission' (ibid.). The idea of 'listening to someone' implies sensitivity to his or her needs and desires. Again, an acoustic practice is used to reference a compassionate mode of attention. With due acknowledgment of the need to avoid carelessly conflating 'listening' and 'hearing' as ways of engaging with sound, it is clear that Kirsch reconfirms the association between hearing and affect identified in the audiovisual litany provided by Sterne. The auditory nature of auscultation is used to naturalize its association with the sympathetic and empathetic elements of medical work.

In the discourse of the death of the stethoscope, then, a set of sensory assumptions as to the nature of auscultation as an auditory technique and echocardiography as a visual one are being used to make arguments as to how medicine should be practised, and what kind of person a doctor should be. Some of the arguments urging the importance of auscultation are arguably flavoured by a kind of idealization of and nostalgia for a type of medical practice that is perceived to be disappearing or under threat. But they also represent an effort to resist or warn of the potential consequences of a more dominant drive towards investment in technology within Western medicine. As the chapter has explained, this drive is in turn linked to an underlying cultural conviction that vision represents the proper sensory route to the acquisition of objective clinical knowledge. Sensory politics, then, is fundamental to debates surrounding medical technology and its integration into medical practice. The senses, and notions of their inherent nature, are used to motivate movement toward change, stasis and even regression in medical culture.

I have described in Chapter 4 how the stethoscope as an icon of medical identity is used in the movements, gestures and routines that in turn articulate a medical 'habitus'. The manner in which many doctors engage in a conspicuous display of the stethoscope and the ways in which the instrument is handled and applied by individual users can be seen to articulate relative levels of professional seniority and skill. But this chapter has sought to open up the medical profession's relationship with the stethoscope more broadly. In the discourse of the death of the stethoscope the instrument has come to stand for an ideal, a way of working and being in which the doctor practises as a skilled but also sensitive and socially resourceful individual. Perhaps it is because the stethoscope has come to signify the doctor's value as a highly technically trained yet intuitive professional that some doctors cling so closely to these instruments and seem so keen to exhibit them on both the wards and corridors of the hospital. That value is something of which they are keen to remind not only their patients and colleagues, but also themselves.

CONCLUSION

In May 2011 I was invited to give a Perspective Tour of the permanent collection at the Wellcome Museum in London. At the entrance to this collection there was (and still is at the time of writing) a set of tall open shelves housing an impressive range of glassware including huge jars and items of laboratory equipment. On the day of the tour I asked the audience to visualize themselves knocking over these shelves or hurling the pieces of glassware to the ground, whilst thinking of the extraordinary crashing, shattering and tinkling of glass they would produce. I made the point that sound recording was in its infancy at the time Henry Wellcome was building his collection, so that thinking about the sounds that the objects in it would have produced, or that might have accompanied their use, requires imagination. I also suggested that the history of medicine would surely have been noisy. An acoustic archaeology of medicine would evoke a vast and terrifying cacophony of wheezing, sneezing, coughing, shivering, screams of pain, sighs of relief and so on. I asked the tour audience to imagine these sounds bursting, seeping and dripping out of the glass containers as they smashed.

Moving beyond this very generalized sonic history, I asked the audience to think more specifically about some of the individual objects on display. Could they imagine the soft shuffling sounds made by the moccasins believed to have belonged to Florence Nightingale as she walked the wards of the Scutari military hospital? Or the pleas for help that preceded the bestowal of healing touches from the silver-mounted lodestone reputed to have been used by Queen Anne? Or the shrieks accompanying the pulling of the teeth now dangling from the Chinese doctor's signboard? Historians interested in the sounds of the past have developed more systematic and rigorous responses to the challenge of 'un-air[ing] sounds that have faded' (Smith 2003:129). This book, however, has gone some way towards showing that the medical cacophony is ongoing. Sound remains an important aspect of many illness experiences and continues to be appropriated in efforts to understand the body, investigate disease and circulate medical information. The book might be understood as an effort to unravel or tease apart a particular medical cacophony, isolating specific ways in which, on the wards studied, sounds are produced and become endowed with meaning through the listening practices of patients and medical professionals. The study is not, of course, an entirely comprehensive investigation of the auditory culture of the hospital, and this conclusion outlines potentially productive directions for future research. It also includes some reflection on research methodology, indicating ways in which auscultation, a key focus of the book, might be valuable as an ethnographic as well as a clinical technique. Finally, the discussion indicates how the concept of 'the body' provides a unifying theme linking the topics covered and points made in the book as a whole.

Considerations for future study

The focus in this ethnography has been on diagnostic and monitory listening and on patient responses to the soundscape of the cardiothoracic wards at St Thomas' Hospital in particular. But there are other environments within the hospital, too, in which specialized listening techniques are employed and particular sounds become laden with significance. In the Intensive Care Unit, for instance, where patients who are very seriously ill are given close medical attention, the use of medical technologies is particularly heavy. Equipment there produces a considerable range of tones, alarms and other sounds to which staff must remain attentive, meaning that monitory listening practices are clearly in evidence. The same applies to the Recovery Room, where patients are taken immediately after surgery. During my research several nurses described to me how patients under the influence of anaesthetic drugs and strong painkillers often have hallucinations or vivid dreams into which the equipment, its lights and particularly its sounds become incorporated. Indeed, noise in ITU's (Intensive Treatment Units) has been linked to a phenomenon called ITU Psychosis whereby patients may experience a range of disturbances, including hearing voices or becoming paranoid and disoriented. A study of the auditory experience of patients in the ITU promises much in terms of developing one of the key concerns of this book, namely the unexpected associations, flights of imagination and fantasy which can be stimulated by the sounds of medical technologies and which sometimes become closely involved in patients' experiences of illness and of their own bodies.

On maternity wards, the sounds of women in labour and of babies crying are particularly marked. Midwives and doctors must also pay close auditory attention to the heartbeat of the foetus. To what extent are electronic monitoring techniques replacing foetal auscultation? Has foetal ultrasound rendered obsolete the use of the Pinard stethoscope (which was designed for listening to the heartbeats of babies in the womb)? It would also be fascinating to know whether medical professionals are sensitive to different tones or notes in the cries of women during labour or in those of newborns. Although, to my knowledge, maternity wards have yet to receive attention from those working within sound studies, this medical environment represents a particularly promising area for future study and offers further insight (or perhaps insound would be a more appropriate term) into connections between listening, the body, health, illness and personhood.

As suggested in Chapter 4, my research was conducted prior to the introduction of smartphones and therefore does not include detailed consideration of how applications such as the iStethoscope Pro have impacted on the way that auscultation is practised and taught in hospitals in the present day. I hope that the research included in this book will be re-appraised by future researchers working in contexts where the iStethoscope Pro is in use. I understand, for instance, that Karin Bijsterveld, Professor of Technology & Society Studies at Maastricht University, is currently leading a project entitled *Sonic Skills: Sound and Listening in Science, Technology and Medicine, 1920s-now*, which will include ethnographic research into how auscultation is practised on the wards of a hospital in the Netherlands. The findings of this study will no doubt detail the use of recent technological innovations relating to auscultation. Research into sonic skills in a Netherlands hospital also promises to create a comparative perspective on aspects of the discussion presented here, and invites further comparative studies to explore the sonic knowledge practices found in hospitals in non-Western settings.

Work from within 'sound studies' has explored uses of sound and listening in institutional environments including schools and detention centres. This study has sought to break new ethnographic ground by exploring the auditory culture of the hospital. However, it also points to the need for ethnographic studies to engage with other institutional environments. For instance, though research has explored many aspects of the experience of imprisonment, the significance of the distinctive soundscapes of prisons for prisoners and staff is currently totally unstudied. My own preliminary research has shown that in an environment where inmates spend much of their time confined to cells and where walls and corridors mean they are frequently unable to gain a visual perspective on their surroundings, sounds can convey important information, announce the imminence of activities, mark events and carry news. Attention to the sonic environment may also be useful to prison staff, informing them of the mood of prisoners, alerting them to potential dangers or incidents. As Chapter 2 indicates is the case on hospital wards, listening may also be a key strategy of surveillance and control inside prisons. Further research is needed to gain a full understanding of the auditory cultures of prisons among other institutions.

It might be pointed out that despite its attempt to discuss and describe a realm of vivified and animate sound, this book is in fact made up of a set of still, silent visual surfaces. Peek points out that media have been available for some time that allow recorded sound to be included alongside or inside text, stating: '[t]he technology is available to augment the silence of print' (1994:489). Digital media have meant that this statement is now truer than ever, and Peek is arguably quite correct when he states that '[w]e should no longer accept "silent" publications on sound' (ibid.:488). Sound recordings can be of great value both illustratively and analytically, and publications are increasingly finding ways to connect text and audio (e.g. Pinch and Bijsterveld 2012, Hume 2008). Sound compositions, too, offer a promising form of ethnographic representation that remains to be fully explored. But though there may be considerable benefits in linking recorded sound to anthropological texts, thereby producing an anthropology 'in' as well as 'on' or 'about' sound, in this book sounds are represented in words alone (Feld and Brenneis 2004).

It could be claimed that sound and sonic experience suffer particularly badly when translated into text because, as Murch suggests and as was indicated in Chapter 5, Western society in particular has never developed an appropriate vocabulary to describe or otherwise cope with the heard world (1994:xvi-xvii). This seems to me, however, to be a somewhat defeatist position that disregards the vocabulary Western society does have for engaging with sound. At the same time, although I acknowledge the difficulty of representing the heard world verbally, I am not persuaded of the fundamental incapacity of the text to convey sonic presences and experiences adequately. Indeed, some anthropological writing is extremely strong in its evocation and description of sound and sonic meaning (Turnbull 1961, Feld 1996, Chuengsatiansup 1999). This is also true of certain works of literary fiction (Ballard [1971] 2001, Conrad [1897] 1987, Calvino 2001, McGregor 2003). Much as I embrace the prospect of an anthropology 'in' sound, then, I think anthropologists should not consider that writing about auditory phenomena and experience is an inherently flawed or failed endeavour, or at least, if it is so, they should find and emphasize what is gained and retained as well as lost in ethnographic translation. Recordings and compositions should, in my view, be incorporated into ethnographic texts and, where justified, even be regarded as ethnographic documents in their own right. Listening and recording should be given the same authority and value as reading and writing within the academic establishment. At the same time, though, adept and insightful writing on sound is still necessary, useful and precious. As well as re-stating the claim that recordings and compositions are important to the realization of a 'sounded anthropology', anthropologists should do all they can to represent sound effectively in their texts (Samuels *et al.* 2010). An absence of recordings should not in itself affect the value of this or any other ethnographic work on sound.

Methodology

In his introduction to William Carlos Williams' book *The Doctor Stories*, Robert Coles refers to 'the busy doc who yet could be spellbound by what he chanced to hear, and knew to keep in mind at night when the typewriter replaced the stethoscope as his major professional instrument' (1984:xi). I am interested in Coles' juxtaposition of these two objects. During fieldwork at St Thomas' they became my professional instruments too. I do not pretend that I had any of the skill which Williams brought to his work with either of them, but my fieldwork was also often a question of putting down one and picking up the other.

Throughout my study at the Edinburgh Royal Infirmary the patients to whom I spoke had generally been in hospital for long periods. Many were bored, waiting for tests, procedures or improvements in their health that would allow them to go home. They were happy to talk to me, often for hours when they had no visitors, and I could reasonably expect that they would be found in the same beds on the same wards for several consecutive days. Conversations could be left and picked up, paused and continued. St Thomas', though, was a bigger, busier hospital. I still encountered some patients who had been there for a long time and who were waiting for tests and operations or for the dates of tests and operations to be fixed so that they could begin waiting for them. Most, though, tended not to stay on the wards of the cardiothoracic unit for long. A patient I spoke to one morning might be gone, either home or moved to a different ward, the same afternoon. Others, brought to St Thomas' from a distance, might stay for one night and then be transferred back to their local hospitals until their operation date. It seemed to be unclear to anyone, particularly the patients themselves, exactly how long they would stay in one place. For me as a fieldworker there was a semblance of chaos that was in fact a complex network of schedules and timeframes negotiated between different authorities within the hospital.

The working environment at St Thomas' was also fast-paced. Though the medical students were under relatively little time pressure and did a good deal of 'hanging around' both in and outside the hospital, for the doctors there was a constant need to move forward, to keep up, to hurry. While happy for me to accompany them on ward rounds or attend consultations, owing to time constraints they were unwilling to schedule meetings for interviews. Though keen to chat before a lecture or grab a coffee afterwards, they were reluctant to create space in their timetables for conversation. I began to realize that trying to work against the pace I encountered would be like trying to paddle against a strong current, and that my methods would have to fit into the working patterns of the doctors. A methodology based around long periods of sustained interaction would not work. Instead, it must involve brief yet focused moments of contact. Considering this I was struck by the analogy of auscultation. The use of the stethoscope almost invariably involves short interactions, fleeting spells of intense concentration and careful, considered listening; my research would require the same.

The practice of auscultation connects people, usually doctors and patients but also students and teaching doctors as well as students and other students as they collaborate in trying to create a shared understanding of particular body sounds. The tubes of the stethoscope served to trace a network of social connections through which auscultation as a skill was transmitted. Illuminating these traces was central to my ethnographic practice in the hospital, and in some ways I could simply follow the stethoscopes. Other features of stethoscopic listening also seemed to create interesting links with fieldwork. Auscultation involves a tension between proximity and distance. The technique requires doctor and patient to get close to one another, but also ensures that there is a degree of separation between them. In ethnographic fieldwork, ethnographer and protagonist also come into close contact, while the ethnographer tries to keep some reflexive distance on the situation in which he or she is involved. In addition, the balance of subjectivity (in the experience of sounds) and objectivity (in constituting those sounds as perceptual objects about which rational judgments may be made) that occurs in auscultation offers a parallel to the balance of subjectivity and objectivity that defines the conduct of successful ethnography. Auscultation, it seemed, could provide the methodological template for, as well as the object of, my research. In certain ways auscultation suggested itself as a way of allowing itself to be examined. The stethoscope might act as a conceptual model for fieldwork. It might be intellectually constructive 'to follow the adventures of its metaphors' (Ellman 1993:15).

In the Introduction I commented on the concept of the 'ethnographic ear'. The fact that much of my research centred on cardiac auscultation suggested to me that it might be possible to refine my particular understanding of the ethnographic ear and perhaps, with tongue slightly in cheek, think in terms of the 'stethnographic ear'. In Chapter 4 I engaged with some of the affordances offered to doctors and medical students by the stethoscope as an instrument.

It seemed, however, that the stethoscope could also offer affordances to the anthropologist conducting fieldwork. Of course, auscultation all too easily becomes a metaphor for getting at things below the surface. It could be used to refer to an effort to understand the inner workings of social life through concentrated auditory attention on the part of the ethnographer, to diagnose societal issues or probe social relations. But as I have indicated, auscultation seems to provide something more solid than a metaphor or an opportunity for navel-listening. It provided, in my own research setting at least, an indication of how to engage with the hospital setting at a practical level whilst also serving as an 'epistemologically provocative model for how researchers can take sound seriously' (Feld and Brenneis 2004:61). I would suggest that other anthropologists might consider the manner in which the sonic practices, objects and technologies with which they engage also offer methodological affordances.

Sound, listening and the body

It has been suggested by psycho-acousticians that a large proportion of sounds that originate within the body are screened out by the ear. This is necessary in order for the outside world to be audible (Barany 1938, Tonndorf 1972). Otherwise, as Ackerman suggests, 'the sounds of our own bodies might be as deafening as sitting in a lawn chair next to a waterfall' (1990:189). Using the same watery metaphor, Carpenter and McLuhan suggest that the ears filter out 'the continuous Niagara of sound...in the circulation of the blood' (1960:68). This book, however, represents an effort both consciously to unlearn insensitivity to the sounds of the body as lived and to draw attention to the wider sonic potentials of the body. Chapter 3 noted that Laennec first improvized a stethoscope by rolling up a stack of paper and pressing it to his patient's chest. This book might also be thought of as a stethoscopic stack of paper, directing auditory attention towards the body with the aim of effecting the amplification of its acoustic possibilities.

In Chapter 7 I introduced Henriques' concept of the 'sonic body', which he suggests 'implies either and both the body of the sound and the sound of the body' (2003:471–2). A related idea is put forward by Brown, who refers to the 'aural body' (2010:214). Brown writes that in hearing, the body produces an 'organic, sympathetically resonant response to external, air-based acoustic energy', but he states that 'the aural body is also a sonic instrument' (ibid.). Some of the sounds that are produced by the body, such as vocal sounds or clapping, are generally deliberate and voluntary. Others, however, are involuntary, and Brown describes 'the personal soundscape of one's own breathing, wheezing, rumbling, swallowing, sniffing, coughing and so on' which one continually inhabits (ibid.). Brown, then, indicates that the body is simultaneously sonically receptive, voluntarily and involuntarily sonically productive and also receptive of its own sonic productivity. This book also emphasizes the multi-dimensional aurality of the body and has explored some of the ways in which, within the hospital, these aural facets might be understood to interact.

Brown makes repeated reference to the medieval concept of *musica humana*, where 'physiological and psychological health depended on a harmonic balance between the various energy centres and important organs of the body, much as the health of the cosmos – *musica mundana* – depended on harmonic relationships between the spheres' (ibid.:134). During fieldwork I found that doctors in the cardiothoracic unit, while not concerned with harmonic balance per se, were often working to restore the normal rhythms of the heart. This was most obvious when medication or a procedure known as 'cardioversion therapy' was used to correct arrhythmia in a patient's heartbeat. A concern with restoring normal sounds also became apparent in the treatment of heart murmurs. For instance, on one occasion at an outpatient clinic Dr Coltart was reviewing a woman who had undergone heart valve surgery three months previously. Having listened to her chest Dr Coltart said 'Well, before the surgery I used to be able to hear a murmur there, and now I can't hear one any more, so I know that you're better and the problem's gone.' Similarly, in the transcript given in Chapter 4 of the *City Hospital* appearance made by Dr Coltart, the firm of students and myself, we hear Dr Coltart explain that the murmur that can be heard in Mary's chest may disappear when her heart muscle picks up following bypass surgery, so that the murmur has been heard 'for the last time maybe'. The abnormal sound will disappear when the heart function improves. Of course, the cardiologist's concern is generally with effecting electrochemical or physiological changes rather than seeking to redress the balance between energy centres and organs in the body. Also, there is no indication that it is by correcting sounds alone that balance within the body is restored, or that correcting sounds is all that is required in order for a problem to be resolved. Rather, the normalization of acoustic signs is one of the consequences of a return to healthy function. Nonetheless, the notion that a healthy body will sound healthy, or that a healthy-sounding body is a healthy body, does resonate with the concept of *musica humana*. Perhaps we could say that in contemporary medical practice, *musica humana* becomes more literal than is implied by the abstract concern with bodily harmony apparent in the medieval sense of the term. The modern *musica humana* consists of actual rhythms and sounds that are heard in the body through diagnostic listening or that are generated by medical equipment in response to the body.

Fundamentally concerned with theatre practice, Brown suggests that '[t]he aural body is the intimate theatre we live in, and all wider theatres are experienced through it' (ibid.:215). He indicates that the aural body is something we inhabit and which inhabits us, but which also mediates our experiences of the soundscapes in which we become immersed and through which we move. This book, too, illustrates that while the body is acoustically sensitive, listening is not only a process through which information is gathered about external environments. Sounds are also generated and perceived to originate from inside the body, produced by its material processes. They are an aspect of corporeality.

Giving a historical overview of the use of listening in medical techniques of examination, Chapter 3 drew attention to the diversity of sounds produced by the animate body. While it appears that medical practitioners have for centuries loosely indexed certain of these sounds to underlying corporeal events and processes, following the anatomical turn and the emergence of modern medicine the bodies of sick patients underwent a more intensive acoustic interrogation. The stethoscope enabled fine distinctions to be drawn between sounds that, through the subsequent autopsy of dead patients, were referenced to specific underlying corporeal states and pathologies. The dark bodily interior underwent a gradual acoustic illumination, becoming increasingly intelligible to listening medical practitioners. Through diagnostic listening techniques and in particular auscultation, the body was constituted in medicine as an object that could be known and explored through its sounds. Stethoscopic listening tapped into and exploited the sonic productivity of the body.

Brown's notion that the body is itself a sonic space nesting within larger sonic spaces is particularly relevant to the material covered in this book. On the wards the bodies of patients (themselves, as indicated above, acoustically intelligible to doctors through auscultation) were also, to borrow from Ingold (2006), 'ensounded', immersed in the distinctive institutional sound environment of the hospital. But a striking feature of the soundscapes of wards on the cardiothoracic unit in particular was the diversity of ways in which bodies were made sonically present within them. This occurred in part simply through the voluntary and involuntary vocalizations and physical movements that were made by patients, visitors, nurses, doctors and other medical professionals. But information about bodily processes and events was also broadcast and circulated through sound in the form of medical discourse and in the signals produced by medical technologies used in diagnosis and monitoring. The body undergoes numerous processes of sonic articulation on the wards and is made acoustically present in a diversity of ways.

Interior corporeal events and processes were externalized through sound on the cardiothoracic wards in particular. This might be understood to happen with auscultation, in which the patient's interior body sounds are brought out into the perception of the listening doctor. But in this case only the doctor is party to the goings on within the patient body. The physiological processes sonified and amplified by diagnostic or monitoring technologies, however, project into public acoustic and discursive space. Sounds spill or seep from patients who in turn sense their bodies being rendered porous and permeable. The body becomes fluid rather than self-contained, creating an 'unbounded' corporeal spatiality (Lawton 1998). For patients, this loss of auditory control over their own bodies, and the encroachment of sounds originating from or produced by other patients in close proximity, may not only emphasize a loss of privacy brought about by entry into an institutional environment but may also present a challenge to the maintenance of individual corporeal integrity. A consideration of ward soundscapes destabilizes the notion that the body is tightly bounded and contained. Sound brings about a dramatic reconfiguration of normal bodily boundaries, even causing the body to be turned, acoustically, inside out.

In the hospital setting the body becomes the object of modes of listening and sonic knowing practised on the one hand by trained doctors, nurses and other medical professionals, and on the other, by untrained patients. We can see medical professionals using listening, for instance, to effect an acoustic objectification of particular sounds and the body parts or physiological states to which they correspond. Not generally possessing the 'auditus eruditus' of those responsible for their care in hospital, patients are usually obliged to listen with less educated and informed ears (Nicolson 2004:157). As a consequence, overhearing for example the technological sounds of echocardiography and electrocardiography, patients may find themselves in the disconcerting situation of effectively eavesdropping on their own bodies, leaving themselves prone to interpreting sounds in ways which stimulate anxieties and even provoke disturbing fantasies or unwelcome incursions into their psychic as well as corporeal integrity. By drawing on Mol (2002), the book has suggested that sounds may become involved in both professional and lay ways of 'doing' disease, thus becoming an element of the distinct 'versions' of the body which, she indicates, coexist in the hospital setting and produce the 'body multiple'.

Reflecting on the sounds of his own body, Brown writes: 'I have largely learned to be deaf to my own constant noise, only becoming aware of it at moments when I am alone or silent' (2010:215). While our own bodies may be generally quiet to us, Chapter 7 introduced the practice of auto-auscultation in which both patients and medical students became acutely conscious of their own heart sounds. This, for the students, was part of learning to auscultate and, while often conducted playfully, was directed towards their attaining familiarity with auscultation and acquiring a firm understanding of the relationship of the heart sounds to the cardiac cycle. Guided by doctors, however, patients were brought to interpret the sounds they heard as indicators of underlying disease. They were led to match their suffering to an audible cause. Auto-auscultation became a serious and significant affair. For a few patients whose heart sounds were unusually loud and were audible without the mediation of the stethoscope, sounds became directly linked to sensations of 'feeling' and 'being' unwell. They were part of the bodily 'dys-appearance', the lived manifestation of disease itself (Leder 1990:69). Thus, the practice of auto-auscultation highlights the fact that the body may be both an object of knowledge and a locus of experience. It also draws attention to complexities of the sonically productive and receptive body simultaneously 'mediating' and 'being' our experience in the world.

Above it was suggested that patients and medical professionals generally have differing knowledge and experience of how to attend to and attribute meaning to the sounds they encounter on the wards. Yet the example of auto-auscultation in particular shows medical students and patients to be involved in fundamentally similar efforts to locate and interpret the clinical significance of sounds from within the body. There is also a broadly similar awareness of sonic embodiment for all listeners, be they students or patients, providing a unification of medical and lay experience. But the differences of perspective between (generally healthy, medically trained) students and (generally sick, medically untrained) patients cannot be altogether ignored, so that the research overall reveals an interesting tension between the singularity and multiplicity of the body in the clinical setting. Rather than resolving this tension one way or the other by unreservedly embracing or rejecting Mol's assertion that multiple ontologies of the (heard or sounded) body co-exist within the hospital, I prefer to leave the tension hanging in the air. To do otherwise would be to misrepresent the ambiguity of the 'sonic' or 'aural' body as it was manifested on the wards.

Pinch and Bijsterveld draw a distinction between 'monitory listening', which they suggest is generally used to determine whether something is wrong, and 'diagnostic listening', which is used to ascertain what is wrong (2012b:14). In my research, both monitory and diagnostic listening are shown to be prevalent on the wards studied. Both modes of auditory attention are used in the surveillance of the patient body, evaluating and re-evaluating its condition relative to a set of clinical concepts and criteria of normalcy. As shown in Chapter 1, however, monitory listening is also integral to the surveillance carried out by nurses as they gauge the atmosphere of the ward and alert themselves to signs of unusual or unacceptable behaviour among patients whom they are supervising. In their monitory listening, then, nurses carry out surveillance not only of the individual corporeal patient body, but also of a wider social grouping, the 'body of patients' or 'patient body' that they must manage and oversee. Monitory listening is centrally involved in ensuring that patients follow the regulations and routines of the wards on which they are staying. As Foucault (1973) suggests, surveillance is orientated towards the production of obedient, docile bodies. Monitory listening, then, is used to manage both patients' internal, involuntary bodily states and the attitudes and actions that constitute their externalized behaviour on the ward.

Nurses might not receive formal training in monitory listening, but their work demands that they be, to some extent at least, sensitive and responsive to those sounds on the ward that serve as indicators as to when and where attention is needed. This book has described in detail, however, how medical students are obliged to undergo formal training in auscultation as part of the process of becoming doctors. They learn to handle and apply the stethoscope in an appropriate manner, gradually acquiring familiarity with sounds that have been identified as holding value as diagnostic signs. In medical training, the sonic receptivity of student bodies is channelled, directed, trained and modified. It is honed so as to create a specialist appreciation of both the sonically productive 'patient body' as an abstract field of knowledge and of the palpably 'real' material bodies medical students and doctors encounter on the wards.

Chapter 4 drew on Sinclair's (1997) description of the medical habitus to identify a specific set of dispositions which structure the way in which doctors think and act. It indicated that, as they undergo their medical education, students adopt or internalize these dispositions, reproducing them in their own patterns of thought and action as they work within their chosen profession. The chapter suggested that the medical habitus is partly acquired through students' imitation of the professional mannerisms and gestures they observe in qualified doctors around them. By drawing on the habitus concept, then, the discussion again foregrounds the body, and specifically the medical student body, as an analytic concern, this time positioning it as a site for the reproduction of the set of schemes for thought and action that characterize the medical habitus.

The book has pointed to the inadequacy of the habitus as a framework for engaging with the intricacies of sensory knowledge. It also critiques the tendency toward the homogenization of bodies (and therefore of sensory abilities) that is implicit within the habitus concept. The notion of habitus has proved useful, however, firstly in situating listening as an embodied, corporeal practice and secondly in highlighting how practice is involved in the development of identities. Thus it was suggested that stethoscopic listening presents an opportunity for students to perform what they consider to be an archetypal medical, or rather 'doctorly' set of gestures, allowing them neatly to express the key dispositions of the medical habitus. Stethoscopic listening initiates a bodily performance of conscientiousness and competency, indeed, an entire professional demeanour. The stethoscope can be regarded as a cultural apparatus or material artefact whose agency is harnessed by medical students in constructing their changing identity, precipitating a transition towards 'doctorhood'.

In a similar way, senior doctors are expected to be able to auscultate quickly and decisively. This is especially true on the cardiothoracic unit where cardiologists are frequently required to make decisions as to the character and significance of subtle heart sounds. At the same time, mastery in auscultation could serve as an index of a doctor's more general medical skill, his command of and confidence in clinical situations. The practice was bound up in the expression and reproduction of the professional hierarchy, being a means by which senior doctors articulated their status and authority on the hospital wards. But Chapter 8 also showed how auscultation can be a technique through which doctors recognize and feel themselves to be a particular kind of medical professional: one that is skilled, resourceful, knowledgeable and valued. Indeed, it was suggested that the stethoscope has been adopted by some doctors as a symbol of this way of working and being. One of the reasons that the prospect of the 'death of the stethoscope' is so troubling is that it threatens the demise of a cherished form of personhood.

To end where this study began, Chapter 1 emphasized that ward soundscapes play an important role for patients in marking, establishing and reinforcing the institutional character of the hospital. It was partly by listening to the sounds of the ward that patients initially came to recognize and then were persistently reminded of their situation within a system of medical work. It was suggested that the soundscape plays a role in forcing patients to recognize their 'patienthood', so that we see the emergence of a sonically ordered sense of self, a 'selfhood' shaped by sound. On the hospital wards in which I conducted fieldwork, then, sound and ways of listening are shown to be integral to the construction not only of bodies, but also of persons.

APPENDIX

The Doctor

The ticking of the clock was infuriating. Dr Francis narrowly overcame his urge to hurl it against the wall, smashing it to smithereens. Instead he snatched it off the bedside table and slid it under the pillow. The metronomic beat, though, refused to be smothered. He could still hear the tiny scratches of the second hand, each tick like the stroke of a pencil crossing through another second of his life. Dr Francis felt the palms of his hands grow sweaty and an angry breath hissed out from between his clenched teeth. He pulled the clock out from under the pillow and carried it downstairs. Opening the airing cupboard he sandwiched it between two towels. He could no longer hear the ticking, but he still felt tense, listless. He was like a rabbit's ear, alert and nervous, twitching first one way, then another, never settling.

The doctor listened to himself complain. He was tired. He hadn't slept well. Noises in the night had kept him awake. The house was old and it creaked and bumped like a shipwreck. The floorboards moaned to one another. The windows were a fraction loose in their wooden frames and banged whenever the slightest breeze blew; then the draught made the drapes rustle like a snake in leaves. Her lateness was not helping. It must be half past eleven by now and still no sign! He became conscious of the sound of his own heart thumping.

Dr Francis scurried back upstairs to check once again that everything was in place. The bed linen looked clean and was neatly turned down and he pulled at the curtains once again to shut out the tiny crack of light which had appeared between them. On the bedside table were fifty pounds in crisp notes, and there, draped over the wardrobe door, were his stethoscopes. He had spent the best part of the morning polishing them, and now he saw their cold metallic gleam in the half-light of the darkened room. Picking up the Littman

II, he felt the rubbery flex of the tubing. It had an elastic, muscular feel. It was strong and supple. The stethoscopes reassured him. They filled him with a strange confidence.

It was at medical school that Dr Francis had first become hypnotized by the stethoscope. The same day that he and his classmates had bought their shiny new instruments, his peers took to wearing them across their white-coated shoulders as if modelling them for catwalk photographers. But they had no idea how to use them, no concept of the stethoscope's power or the new sight it might bestow upon the skilled user. Dr Francis had realized its potential immediately. He spent hours each evening reading textbooks, listening to his own heart, learning the points at which its sounds might be heard the clearest, familiarizing himself with the intricacies of its rhythm, the extremities of its resonance, the heart beat's gentle acceleration when he took a deep breath, its deceleration when he let it out.

One day the professor had made all the members of his class listen to one another's chests, just to familiarize themselves with the first and second heart sounds, the lub-dup rhythm. Dr Francis, then just plain Anthony, had been paired with Jessica, the most beautiful girl in the firm. Sliding his hand under her jumper and feeling it move with the rise and fall of her chest had been pleasant enough. But the sensation was insignificant compared to the thrill of detecting the quiet click of a mitral valve prolapse in late systole – the valve sound slightly thicker, with the unmistakable click, like the sound of an earring being gently placed on a glass-topped dressing table. He had chosen not to tell about the clicking, thinking it best to pretend everything was normal, but he carried the secret around with him and re-played it time after time in his head.

Dr Francis had loved what he enjoyed referring to as 'auscultation', a highfalutin term for listening with a stethoscope. He was a natural at it. While his classmates had often had to lie, nodding unconvincingly when the consultant asked them if they had heard, for instance, the pan-systolic murmur of mitral regurgitation, Dr Francis would colour in the basic terminology, elaborating using adjectives like 'musical' or 'rumbling'. He would surprise his superiors with strikingly pertinent questions, such as 'Does the mitral turbulence influence blood pressure in the pulmonary vein?' or 'Would one expect to find a complementary malar flush?' As the others struggled with the basic ejection-systolic murmur of aortic stenosis, Dr Francis could reliably detect a gallop rhythm or even isolate the shunting sound produced by a septal defect. The professor had recognized his exceptional ability, and advised him to specialize as a cardiologist. It had been good advice. He passed the exams with flying colours, and thereafter enjoyed, no, loved almost every day of his working life. To him cardiology was not just his work. It was his passion.

The doctor's reverie was interrupted by a scratch at the glass of the French windows. 'At last!' Dr Francis said out loud. He hurried back downstairs. Pulling back the curtain he tried not to look at the girl through the glass doors, preferring to keep his head bowed and to stare down at his hands as they fiddled with the lock. Finally he slid the door open. A breath of cold, fresh air swept past him into the house like an energetic dog. Dr Francis stood, still and silent. There was a long pause.

'I can't stay long,' said the girl finally. 'You've got half an hour.'

The doctor didn't move. There was another long pause.

'I suppose it would be best if you came upstairs,' he said at last.

The girl nodded, and followed him up the staircase.

The doctor did not turn to face her as they entered the bedroom, nor did he as he spoke to her. 'Just take off your top things and lie on the bed,' he instructed.

Giving her time to undress he walked over to the wardrobe. The tubes of his three stethoscopes dangled down over the mirror on the inside of the door. The sight of them filled him with intense pride and excited anticipation. He picked up the Allen Gemini with its old-fashioned dual conductor tubing and heavy alloy headpiece. This had accompanied him on ward rounds for many years. He had listened to thousands of hearts through it. He felt close to the instrument somehow. It was an old friend, a trusted and respected companion. He was a lesser man without a stethoscope like this one, incompetent and un-resourceful. But as he hung the stethoscope round his neck like a medal he felt a growing sense of control, of mastery even.

Dr Francis heard the rustle of the sheet and the soft gonging of the bedsprings as the girl made herself comfortable. When she seemed to be at rest he turned and walked around to the far side of the bed. As he did so he briefly ran his eyes over her body. A young female in her twenties (he guessed twenty-six) with bright eyes and good colour. Her chest was rising and falling quickly, but evenly and symmetrically. She was, he supposed, beautiful, but her visual characteristics were uninteresting. They were stark and almost vulgar where sounds were subtle and suggestive, implying rather than stating. He studied her left breast. On a reclining woman of this age the left nipple was a good indicator of the apex beat, the point at which the heart sounds of both ventricles could be most easily discerned.

Then, through the twilight of the darkened room, the doctor noticed a dark lesion just below the girl's breast. It stood out as very black against her pale skin. The doctor walked a little closer and peered at the mark. He saw it was not a lesion but a tiny tattoo in dark red ink. Though its edges had softened a little Dr Francis saw that it was a rose – a tiny tattoo of a rose. The girl noticed his interest. 'It seemed like a good idea at the time,' she said and laughed a little nervous laugh. Dr Francis did not return it as he might ordinarily have done. He did not take his eyes off the tiny design. Its position made it exceptional, remarkable. It was exactly where he would place the stethoscope to listen to the heart sounds. 'In a moment, I'm going to listen to that rose,' he told the girl.

He sat on the bed facing away from her, his lower back just touching her hip. He pushed in the earpieces of the stethoscope and the world went muffled. It instantly became distant to him, irrelevant. His attention was directed down the stethoscope towards the girl's body. Normally he would have examined her more carefully for scars or rashes, checked the eyes and tongue, felt the pulse at the wrist. But today there was no need for any of that. He could cut straight to the interesting part. He warmed the diaphragm against the back of his hand for a few seconds, then placed it gently on her chest. She gasped quietly. He closed his eyes, and began to listen.

It was as if his ears had taken a deep breath and were diving. The harsh, sharp sounds of the house which had bothered him for days vanished and floating, watery sounds washed pleasantly into his ears like warm bathwater. There was a loud rushing, brushing sound as the diaphragm settled against her skin. His fingers applied a little pressure, then the rich, boiling throb of her pulse reached him. It was a deeply aquatic experience. Dr Francis sighed and let his ears drink in the sound of her. It was a lovely pulse, a lively andante with a strong, even rhythm of good volume. He let the beat gently insist on itself. Such a sweet sound!

The doctor took his time, something he could not do at the hospital where answers were required quickly, and where lingering over a patient's body might be interpreted as incompetence. He had no one to answer to, no round to make, no instructions to issue or students to teach. The only pressure was blood pressure. The tangle of shirts, vests, bras and jumpers was entirely disposed of. There were no barriers, nothing in the way. He could indulge himself – to his heart's content.

He lifted the stethoscope and traced a path across her chest, pausing to listen from time to time. The stethoscope was like a slug, a leech sucking out sound as if it were blood. Her heart rate accelerated, slightly, but perceptibly. The doctor opened his eyes briefly, watching the diaphragm move over the tiny rose tattoo as if it were a huge moon eclipsing the sun. He pushed the breast tissue up slightly and pressed the diaphragm down against the resistance of her skin. He allowed his ears to hone, deeper than before, trying to make them probe further and further into the horizons of sound which rose to meet him. He closed his eyes tight, trying to redirect the energy from his eyes into his ears, to think himself into his eardrums.

Then suddenly he seemed to clinch, to seize the sound he was seeking out. His ears gathered up the beat, dusting and polishing it until each round thump resonated strongly and colourfully. It was as though someone was beating a huge drum; a clean, powerful sound. This was the beat to which the human race marched, the rhythm to which all life was played out, the sinus rhythm. From Hippocrates to the bag lady at the hospital these beats had underlain all of human experience. They were the fundamental time signature of life. The doctor found no monotony in it. He never grew tired of the sound of a heart beating. There was something primeval about it. Before this girl was born, before she was a person, before she was a soul even, she was this pulsing. Never mind her eyes, her hair, her face – this was her. He was in a place more intimate than even she knew. She herself had never heard and would never hear what he was hearing. It was the very essence of her. The doctor started to drift away, suspended on a tide of sound which dissolved his anxiety, rinsed away the tension which had been building in him for weeks.

'What can you hear?' the girl whispered, so quietly she could hardly even hear her own words. Her voice reached the doctor as if through a dense mist. It had a heavy, breathy quality. He was so suspended in her that he hardly heeded it. 'I can hear *everything*,' he whispered back to her. '*Everything*! It's a beautiful sound! You have a wonderful heart.'

'I'll let myself out, then,' the girl said after a time.

'Forgive me, my dear,' the doctor murmured, his voice heavy with impending slumber. 'I am a slave to my ears.'

'And will you be wanting to *examine* me again?' she asked.

But he didn't hear her. His head had sunk onto the pillow and he was sound asleep. His stethoscope lay like a huge smile across the bed.

This story was first published in *The Erotic Review* 86:74–8. Reproduced with permission.

REFERENCES

Ackerman, D. 1990. *A Natural History of the Senses*. New York: Vintage.

Anderson, C.M.B. and L.S. Whittle. 1971. Physiological Noise and the Missing 6dB. *Acustica* 24:261–72.

Armstrong, D. 1995. The Rise of Surveillance Medicine. *Sociology of Health and Illness* 17(3):393–404.

Atkinson, R. 2006. The Aural Ecology of the City: sound, noise and exclusion in the city. *Occasional Paper No. 5*. Housing and Community Research Unit: University of Tasmania.

Atkinson, R. 2007. Ecology of Sound: the sonic order of urban space. *Urban Studies* 44(10):1905–17.

Attali, J. 1985. *Noise: The Political Economy of Music*. Minneapolis and London: University of Minnesota Press.

Babu, A.N. 1999. Death of the Stethoscope. http://www.acponline.org/journals/news/mar99/letters.htm. Accessed 04/10/2011.

Bachelard, G. [1958] 1994. *The Poetics of Space* (trans. M. Jolas). Boston, Massachusetts: Beacon Press.

Back, L. 2003. Sounds in the Crowd. In *The Auditory Culture Reader* (eds) M. Bull and L. Back, 311–27. Oxford: Berg.

Bailey, P. 1996. Breaking the Sound Barrier: a historian listens to noise. *Body and Society* 2(2):49–66.

Ballard, J.G. [1971] 2001. *Vermilion Sands*. London: Vintage.

Barany, E. 1938. A Contribution to the Physiology of Bone Conduction. *Acta Otolaryngol* 26:1–223.

Bart, S. 2005. The Return of Panopticism: supervision, subjection and the new surveillance. *Surveillance and Society* 3(1):1–20.

Bauman, H.-D.L. 2004. Audism: exploring the metaphysics of oppression. *Journal of Deaf Studies and Deaf Education* 9(2):239–46.

Bauman, H.-D.L. 2008. Listening to Phonocentrism with Deaf Eyes: Derrida's mute philosophy of (sign) language. *Essays in Philosophy* 9:1.

Beer, D. 2010. Mobile music, coded objects and everyday spaces. *Mobilities* 5(4):469–84.

Benthien, C. 2002. *Skin: on the cultural border between self and the world*. New York: Columbia University Press.

Berendt, J. 1983. *The World is Sound: Nada Brahma*. Rochester, Vermont: Destiny Books.

Berger, J. 1967. *A Fortunate Man: the story of a country doctor*. New York: Vintage Books.

Berger, J. 1972. *Ways of Seeing*. London: British Broadcasting Corporation and Penguin Books.

Bharathan, T., D. Glodan, A. Ramesh, B. Vardhini, E. Baccash, P. Kiselev and G. Goldenberg. 2007. What Do Patterns of Noise in a Teaching Hospital and Nursing Home Suggest? *Noise Health* 9:31–4.

Birdsall, C. 2009. Earwitnessing: sound memories of the Nazi period. In *Sound Souvenirs: audio technologies, memory and cultural practice* (eds) K. Bijsterveld and J. van Dijck, 169–81. Amsterdam: Amsterdam University Press.

Bijsterveld, K. 2003. The Diabolical Symphony of the Mechanical Age: technology and symbolism of sound in European and North American noise campaigns, 1900–40. In *The Auditory Culture Reader* (eds) M. Bull and L. Back, 165–89. Oxford: Berg.

Bijsterveld, K. 2008. *Mechanical Sound: technology, culture, and public problems of noise in the twentieth century*. Cambridge, Massachusetts: MIT Press.

Bijsterveld, K. 2010. Acoustic Cocooning: how the car became a place to unwind. *The Senses and Society* 5:189–211.

Blackford, H. 2004. Playground Panopticism: ring-around-the-children, a pocketful of women. *Childhood* 11(2):227–49.

Blesser, B. and L.-R. Salter. 2007. *Spaces Speak, Are You Listening?: experiencing aural architecture*. Cambridge, Massachusetts and London, England. The MIT Press.

Bloch, M. 2008. Truth and Sight: generalizing without universalizing. *Journal of the Royal Anthropological Institute* 14(S1):S22–S32.

Born, G. (ed.) 2013. *Music, Sound and Space: transformations of public and private experience*. Cambridge: Cambridge University Press.

Bourdieu, P. 1977. *Outline of a Theory of Practice* (trans. R. Nice). Cambridge: Cambridge University Press.

Bourdieu, P. 1980. *The Logic of Practice* (trans. R. Nice). Cambridge: Polity.

Bourdieu, P. 1986. *Distinction: a social critique of the judgement of taste* (trans. R. Nice). London: Routledge and Kegan Paul.

Braun, H.-J. 2012. Turning a Deaf Ear?: industrial noise and noise control in Germany since the 1920's. In *The Oxford Handbook of Sound Studies* (eds) T. Pinch and K. Bijsterveld, 58–78. Oxford and New York: Oxford University Press.

Brown, R. 2010. *Sound: a reader in theatre practice*. Basingstoke, Hampshire and New York: Palgrave Macmillan.

Bubandt, N. 1998. The Odour of Things: smell and the cultural elaboration of disgust in Eastern Indonesia. *Ethnos* 63(1):48–80.

Bull, M. 2000. *Sounding Out the City: personal stereos and the management of everyday life*. Oxford and New York: Berg.

Bull, M. and L. Back (eds). 2003a. *The Auditory Culture Reader*. Oxford: Berg.

Bull, M. and L. Back. 2003b. Introduction. In *The Auditory Culture Reader* (eds) M. Bull and L. Back, 1–18. Oxford: Berg.

Bushnell, M. 2003. Teachers in the Schoolhouse Panopticon: complicity and resistance. *Education and Urban Society* 35(3):251–72.

Calvino, I. 2001. *Under the Jaguar Sun*. London: Vintage.

Carpenter, E. 1976. *Oh, What a Blow that Phantom Gave Me!* St Albans: Paladin.

Carpenter, E. and M. McLuhan. 1960. Acoustic Space. In *Explorations in Communication* (eds) E. Carpenter and M. McLuhan, 65–70. Boston: Beacon Press.

Chion, M. 1994. *Audiovision: sound on screen*. New York: University of Columbia Press.

Chuengsatiansup, K. 1999. Sense, Symbol and Soma: illness experience in the soundscape of everyday life. *Culture, Medicine and Psychiatry* 23:272–301.

Classen, C., D. Howes and A. Synnott. 1994. *Aroma: the cultural history of smell*. London and New York: Routledge.

Classen, C. 1998. *The Color of Angels: cosmology, gender and the aesthetic imagination*. London and New York: Routledge.

Classen, C. (ed.) 2005. *The Book of Touch*. Oxford: Berg.

Clifford, J. 1986. Introduction: partial truths. In *Writing Culture: the poetics and politics of ethnography* (eds) J. Clifford and G.E. Marcus, 1–26. Berkeley, Los Angeles and London: University of California Press.

Cohen, E. 2010. Anthropology of Knowledge. *Journal of the Royal Anthropological Institute* (special issue):S193–S202.

Cohen, A.P. and N. Rapport. 1995. Introduction. In *Questions of Consciousness* (eds) A.P. Cohen and N. Rapport, 1–20. London: Routledge.

Coles, R. 1984. Introduction. In *William Carlos Williams: the doctor stories* (ed.) R. Coles, vii-xvi. New York: New Directions.

Connor, S. 1997. The Modern Auditory I. In *Rewriting the Self: histories from the Renaissance to the present* (ed.) R. Porter, 203–23. London: Routledge.

Connor, S. 2000. *Dumbstruck: a cultural history of ventriloquism*. New York: Oxford University Press.

Conrad, J. [1897] 1987. *The Nigger of the 'Narcissus'*. Harmondsworth: Penguin.

Corbin, A. 1994. *The Foul and the Fragrant: odour and the social imagination*. London: Picador.

Corbin, A. 1998. *Village bells: sound and meaning in the nineteenth-century French countryside*. New York: Columbia University Press.

Cox, R. 2006. The Sound of One Hand Clapping: an investigation of the acoustic dimensions of sociality in a Zen temple neighbourhood of Kyoto city, Japan. http://www.st-andrews.ac.uk/soundanth/work/cox/. Accessed 14/01/2012.

Csordas, T.J. 1994. Introduction: the body as representation and being-in-the-world. In *Embodiment and Experience: the existential ground of culture and self* (ed.) T.J. Csordas, 1–26. Cambridge: Cambridge University Press.

Csordas, T.J. 1999. The Body's Career in Anthropology. In *Anthropological Theory Today* (ed.) H. Moore, 172–205. Cambridge: Polity Press.

Cusick, S. 2006. Music as Torture/Music as Weapon. *Transcultural Music Review* 10. http://www.sibetrans.com/trans/a152/music-as-torture-music-as-weapon. Accessed 16/01/2012.

Cusick, S. 2008. 'You Are In a Place Out of the World': music in the detention camps of the 'global war on terror'. *Journal of the Society for American Music* 2:1–27.

Cusick, S. 2013. Toward an acoustemology of detention in the 'global war on terror'. In *Music, Sound, and Space: transformations and public and private experience* (ed.) G. Born, 275–91. Cambridge: Cambridge University Press.

Daniel, V.E. 1991. The Pulse as an Icon in Siddha Medicine. In *The Varieties of Sensory Experience: a sourcebook in the anthropology of the senses* (ed.) D. Howes, 100–10. Toronto, Buffalo and London: University of Toronto Press.

DeNora, T. 2000. *Music in Everyday Life*. Cambridge: Cambridge University Press.

Desjarlais, R. 1992. *Body and Emotion: the aesthetics of illness and healing in the Nepal Himalayas*. Philadelphia: University of Pennsylvania Press.

Downey, G. 2010. 'Practice without Theory': a neuroanthropological perspective on embodied learning. *Journal of the Royal Anthropological Institute* (special issue):S22–S40.

Draper, J. 2002. 'It Was a Real Good Show': the ultrasound scan, fathers, and the power of visual knowledge. *Sociology of Health and Illness* 24(6):771–95.

Drobnick, J. (ed.) 2006. *The Smell Culture Reader*. Oxford: Berg.

Duden, B. 1993. *Disembodying Women: perspectives on pregnancy and the unborn*. Cambridge, Massachusetts: Harvard University Press.

Edwards, E. and K. Bhaumik (eds). 2008. *Visual Sense: a cultural reader*. Oxford: Berg.

Ellman, M. 1993. *The Hunger Artists: starving, writing and imprisonment*. London: Virago.

Erlmann, V. 2004. But What of the Ethnographic Ear? Anthropology, Sound and the Senses. In *Hearing Cultures: essays on sound, listening and modernity* (ed.) V. Erlmann, 1–20. Oxford: Berg.

Fabian, J. 1983. *Time and the Other*. New York: Columbia University Press.
Feld, S. 1990. *Sound and Sentiment: birds, weeping, poetics, and song in Kaluli expression*. Philadelphia: University of Pennsylvania Press.
Feld, S. 1991. Sound as a Symbolic System: the Kaluli drum. In *The Varieties of Sensory Experience: a sourcebook in the anthropology of the senses* (ed.) D. Howes, 79–99. Toronto: University Press.
Feld, S. 1996. Waterfalls of Song: an acoustemology of place resounding in Bosavi, Papua New Guinea. In *Senses of Place* (eds) S. Feld and K.H. Basso, 91–135. Santa Fe: School of American Research Press.
Feld, S. 2003. A Rainforest Acoustemology. In *The Auditory Culture Reader* (eds) M. Bull and L. Back, 223–39. Oxford: Berg.
Feld, S. and D. Brenneis. 2004. Doing Anthropology in Sound. *American Ethnologist* 31:461–74.
Fernandez, J. 1974. The Mission of Metaphor in Expressive Culture. *Current Anthropology* 15:119–45.
Fickers, A. 2012. Visibly Audible: the radio dial as mediating interface. In *The Oxford Handbook of Sound Studies* (eds) T. Pinch and K. Bijsterveld, 411–39. Oxford and New York: Oxford University Press.
Fiddler, G.I., and O. Scott. 1980. Heart Murmurs Audible Across the Room in Children with Mitral Valve Prolapse. *British Heart Journal* 44:201–3.
Fleming, P.R. 1997. *A Short History of Cardiology*. Amsterdam: Rodopi.
Foucault, M. 1973. *The Birth of the Clinic: an archaeology of medical perception* (trans. A.M. Sheridan Smith). New York: Vintage Books.
Foucault, M. 1977. *Discipline and Punish: the birth of the prison* (trans. A.M. Sheridan Smith). New York: Vintage Books.
Foucault, M. 1996. The Eye of Power. In *Foucault Live: collected interviews, 1961–1984* (trans. L. Tochroth and J. Johnston) (ed.) S. Lotringer, 226–40. New York: Semiotext[e].
Fox, R. and J.P. Swazey. 1992. *Spare Parts: organ replacement in American society*. Oxford and New York: Oxford University Press.
Friedson, S.M. 1996. *Dancing Prophets: musical experience in Tumbuka healing*. Chicago: University of Chicago Press.
Furst, L.R. 1998. *Between Doctors and Patients: the changing balance of power*. Charlottesville: University Press of Virginia.
Gallagher, M. 2010. Are Schools Panoptic? *Surveillance and Society* 7(3/4):262–72.
Gallagher, M. 2011. Sound, Space and Power in a Primary School. *Social and Cultural Geography* 12(1):47–61.
Gell, A. 1995. The Language of the Forest: landscape and phonological iconism in Umeda. In *The Anthropology of Landscape: perspectives on place and space* (eds) E. Hirsch and M. O'Hanlon, 232–54. Oxford: Oxford University Press.
Gell, A. 1998. *Art and Agency in Anthropological Theory*. Oxford: Clarendon Press.
Gerchufsky, M. 1995. Ode to a Stethoscope, the Umbilical Cord of Health Care. *Advance* 3:47–50.
Goffman, E. 1968. *Asylums*. Harmondsworth: Penguin.
Goffman, E. 1997. *The Presentation of the Self in Everyday Life*. Harmondsworth: Penguin.
Gonzalez, J.A. 1995. Autotopographies. In *Prosthetic Territories: politics and hypertechnologies* (eds) G. Brahm Jr and M. Driscoll, 133–50. Boulder, California and Oxford: Westview Press.
Good, B.J. 1994. *Medicine, Rationality and Experience: an anthropological perspective*. Cambridge: Cambridge University Press.

Grosz, E. 1992. Voyeurism/exhibitionism/the gaze. In *Feminism and Psychoanalysis: a critical dictionary* (ed.) E. Wright, 449. Oxford: Blackwell Publishers.

Greene, P.D. and T. Porcello. (eds) 2005. *Wired for Sound: engineering and technologies in sonic cultures*. Middletown, Connecticut: Wesleyan University Press.

Gunaratnam, Y. 2009. Auditory Space, Ethics and Hospitality: 'noise', alterity and care at the end of life. *Body and Society* 15:1–19.

Hahn, R.A. 1985. A World of Internal Medicine: portrait of an internist. In *Physicians of Western Medicine: anthropological approaches to theory and practice* (eds) R.A. Hahn and A.D. Gaines, 51–112. Dordrecht, Boston and Lancaster: D. Reidel Publishing.

Haraway, D.J. 1991. *Simians, Cyborgs and Women: the reinvention of nature*. London: Free Association Books.

Haug, M.R. 1988. A Re-Examination of the Hypothesis of Physician Deprofessionalization. *The Millbank Quarterly* 66(2):48–56.

Helmreich, S. 2007. An Anthropologist Underwater: immersive soundscapes, submarine cyborgs, and transductive ethnography. *American Ethnologist* 34(4):621–41.

Henriques, J. 2003. Sonic Dominance and the Reggae Sound System Session. In *The Auditory Culture Reader* (eds) M. Bull and L. Back, 451–80. New York: Berg.

Hirschkind, C. 2006. *The Ethical Soundscape: cassette sermons and Islamic counterpublics*. New York: Columbia University Press.

Hooke, R. 1705. A General Scheme, or Idea of the Present State of Natural Philosophy. In *The Posthumous Works of Robert Hooke* (ed.) R. Waller, 39–40. London: Samuel Smith and Benjamin Walford.

Horning, S.S. 2004. Engineering the Performance: recording engineers, tacit knowledge, and the art of controlling sound. *Social Studies of Science* 34(5):703–31.

Hoskins, J. 1998. *Biographical Objects: how things tell the stories of people's lives*. London and New York: Routledge.

Howes, D. 1988. On the Odour of the Soul: spatial representation and olfactory classification in Eastern Indonesia and Western Melanesia. *Bijdragen* 144:84–113.

Howes, D. 1991a. Introduction: 'to summon all the senses'. In *The Varieties of Sensory Experience: a sourcebook in the anthropology of the senses* (ed.) D. Howes, 3–21. Toronto: University of Toronto Press.

Howes, D. 1991b. Sensorial Investigations. In *The Varieties of Sensory Experience: a sourcebook in the anthropology of the senses* (ed.) D. Howes, 167–91. Toronto: University of Toronto Press.

Howes, D. (ed.) 2009. *The Sixth Sense Reader*. Oxford: Berg.

Howes, D. and C. Classen. 1991. Conclusion: sounding sensory profiles. In *The Varieties of Sensory Experience: a sourcebook in the anthropology of the senses* (ed.) D. Howes, 257–88. Toronto: University of Toronto Press.

Hsu, E. 1999. *The Transmission of Chinese Medicine*. Cambridge: Cambridge University Press.

Hsu, E. 2010. *Pulse Diagnosis in Early Chinese Medicine*. Cambridge: Cambridge University Press.

Hull, J.M. 1990. *Touching the Rock: an experience of blindness*. New York: Pantheon.

Hume, V. (ed.) 2008. *Transplant*. London: rb&hArts.

Ingold, T. 2000. *The Perception of the Environment: essays on livelihood, dwelling and skill*. London: Routledge.

Ingold, T. 2006. Against Soundscape. http://www.st-andrews.ac.uk/soundanth/work/ingold/. Accessed 01/09/2011.

Ingold, T. 2007a. Earth, sky, wind and weather. *Journal of the Royal Anthropological Institute* 13(S1):S19–S38.

Ingold, T. 2007b. Materials against Materiality. *Archaeological Dialogues* 14(1):1–16.

Jackson, J. 1994. Chronic Pain and the Tension between the Body as Subject and Object. In *Embodiment and Experience: the existential ground of culture and self* (ed.) T.J. Csordas, 201–28. Cambridge: Cambridge University Press.

Jenks, C. 1995. The Centrality of the Eye in Western Culture: an introduction. In *Visual Culture* (ed.) C. Jenks, 1–25. London: Routledge.

Johnston, N. 2000. *Forms of Constraint: a history of prison architecture*. Urbana and Chicago: University of Illinois Press.

Jordanova, L. 1989. *Sexual Visions: images of gender in science and medicine between the eighteenth and twentieth centuries*. Wisconsin: University of Wisconsin Press.

Kahn, D. 2001. *Noise, Water, Meat: a history of sound in the arts*. Cambridge, Massachusetts and London: MIT Press.

Kesey, K. 1973. *One Flew Over the Cuckoo's Nest*. London: Picador.

Kirsch, M. 1998. The Death of the Stethoscope: murmurs of discontent. http://www.acponline.org/journals/news/dec98/stetho.htm. Accessed 01/09/2011.

Kittay, J. 2008. The Sound Surround: exploring how one might design the everyday soundscape for the truly captive audience. *Nordic Journal of Music Therapy* 17:41–54.

Kleinman, A. 1995. *Writing at the Margin: discourse between anthropology and medicine*. Berkeley: University of California Press.

Korsmeyer, C. (ed.) 2005. *The Taste Culture Reader*. Oxford: Berg.

Kracauer, S. 1995. *The Mass Ornament: Weimar essays* (trans. T.Y. Levin). Cambridge, Massachusetts: Harvard University Press.

Krebs, S. 2012. 'Sobbing, Whining, Rumbling': listening to automobiles as social practice. In *The Oxford Handbook of Sound Studies* (eds) T. Pinch and K. Bijsterveld, 79–101. Oxford and New York: Oxford University Press.

Labelle, B. 2010. *Acoustic Territories: sound culture and everyday life*: London and New York: Continuum.

Lachmund, J. 1999. Making Sense of Sound: auscultation and lung sound codification in nineteenth-century French and German Medicine. *Science, Technology, and Human Values* 24(4):419–50.

Laderman, C. and M. Roseman (eds). 1996. *The Performance of Healing*. New York and London: Routledge.

Laennec, R.T.H. 1846. *A Treatise on Mediate Auscultation and on Diseases of the Lungs and Heart* (trans. A member of the Royal College of Physicians). London: H. Bailliere.

Lastra, J. 2000. *Sound Technology and the American Cinema: perception, representation, modernity*. New York: Columbia University Press.

Latour, B. 1987. *Science in Action: how to follow scientists and engineers through society*. Milton Keynes: Open University Press.

Latour, B. 1999. *Pandora's Hope: essays on the reality of science studies*. Cambridge, Massachusetts and London: Harvard University Press.

Lave, J. and E. Wenger. 1991. *Situated Learning: legitimate peripheral participation*. Cambridge: Cambridge University Press.

Lawton, J. 1998. Contemporary Hospice Care: the sequestration of the unbounded body and the 'dirty dying'. *Sociology of Health and Illness* 20(2):121–43.

Leach, J. 2003. *Creative Land: place and procreation on the Rai coast of Papua New Guinea*. New York: Berghahn Books.

Leder, D. 1990. *The Absent Body*. Chicago: University of Chicago Press.
Lewis, G. 2000. *A Failure of Treatment*. Oxford: Oxford University Press.
Longmore, M., I. Wilkinson and E. Torok. 2001. *The Oxford Handbook of Clinical Medicine*. Oxford: Oxford University Press.
Lupton, D. 1997. Doctors on the Medical Profession. *Sociology of Health and Illness* 19(4):480–97.
Makovicky, N. 2010. 'Something to Talk About': notation and knowledge-making among central Slovak lace-makers. *Journal of the Royal Anthropological Institute* (special issue):S80–S99.
Mangione, S. 2000. *Physical Diagnosis Secrets*. Philadelphia: Hanley and Belfus.
Mangione, S. and L.Z. Nieman. 1997. New Doctors Have Dangerously Poor Stethoscope Skills. *Journal of the American Medical Association* 278:717–22.
Marchand, T. 2010a. Making Knowledge: explorations of the indissoluble relation between minds, bodies and environment. *Journal of the Royal Anthropological Institute* 2010 (special issue):S1–S21.
Marchand, T. 2010b. Embodied Cognition and Communication: studies with British fine woodworkers. *Journal of the Royal Anthropological Institute* 2010 (special issue):S100–S120.
Margolis, J. 1999. Pierre Bourdieu: habitus and the logic of practice. In *Bourdieu: a critical reader* (ed.) R. Shusterman, 64–83. Oxford: Blackwell.
Marks, G. 1972. *The Story of the Stethoscope*. Folkestone: Bailey and Swinfen.
Markus, T. 1993. *Buildings and Power: freedom and control in the origins of modern building type*. London: Routledge.
Marquez, G.G. 1989. *Love in the Time of Cholera*. Harmondsworth: Penguin.
Matless, D. 2005. Sonic Geography in a Nature Region. *Social and Cultural Geography* 6(5):745–66.
Maulitz, R.C. 1987. *Morbid Appearances: the anatomy of pathology in the early nineteenth century*. New York: Cambridge University Press.
Maurer, C. 2001. Introduction. In *Frederico Garcia Lorca Selected Poems* (ed.) C. Maurer, ix-xx. London: Penguin.
Mauss, M. [1935] 1979. Body techniques. In *Sociology and Psychology: essays by Marcel Mauss* (trans. B. Brewster), 70–87. London: Routledge & Kegan Paul.
McGregor, J. 2003. *If Nobody Speaks of Remarkable Things*. London: Bloomsbury.
McLuhan, M. [1962] 2008. *The Gutenberg Galaxy*. Toronto: University of Toronto Press.
Medical Research Council. 1997. *Report on the Non-Auditory Effects of Noise*. R10.
Miller, D. 2005. Materiality: an introduction. In *Materiality* (ed.) D. Miller, 1–50. Durham: Duke University Press.
Miller, D. 2008. *The Comfort of Things*. London: Polity.
Mody, C.C. 2012. Conversions: sound and sight, military and civilian. In *The Oxford Handbook of Sound Studies* (eds) T. Pinch and K. Bijsterveld, 224–48. Oxford and New York: Oxford University Press.
Mol, A. 2002. *The Body Multiple: ontology in medical practice*. Durham and London, Duke University Press.
Moore, B.C.J. 2003. *An Introduction to the Psychology of Hearing*. London: Academic Press.
Moore, J. 2005. *Cultural Landscapes in the Ancient Andes: archaeologies of place*. Fort Myers: University Press of Florida.
Moran, D. 2000. *Introduction to Phenomenology*. London and New York: Routledge.
Morgan, L. and R. Chambers. 2004. *Enabling Disabled Doctors: a scoping exercise*. Staffordshire University: Disabled Doctors Action Group.

Mulvey, L. 1975. Visual Pleasure and Narrative Cinema. *Screen* 16(3):6–18.
Murch, W. 1994. Foreword. In *Audiovision: sound on screen* (ed.) M. Chion, vii-xxiv. New York: University of Columbia Press.
Nancy, J.-L. 2007. *Listening* (trans. C. Mandell). New York: Fordham University Press.
Nicolson, M. 2004. Having the Doctor's Ear in Nineteenth Century Edinburgh. In *Hearing History: a reader* (ed.) M.M. Smith, 151–186. Athens and London: University of Georgia Press.
Ong, W. 1969. World as View and World as Event. *American Anthropologist* 71(4):634–47.
Ong, W. 1982. *Orality and Literacy: the technologizing of the word.* London and New York: Routledge.
Ong, W. 1991. The Shifting Sensorium. In *The Varieties of Sensory Experience: a sourcebook in the anthropology of the senses* (ed.) D. Howes, 25–30. Toronto: University of Toronto Press.
Osler, W. 1880. On a Remarkable Heart Murmur Heard at a Distance from the Chest Wall. *Medical Times and Gazette, London* II:432–3.
Peek, P. 1994. The Sounds of Silence: cross-world communication and the auditory arts in African societies. *American Ethnologist* 21(3):474–94.
Picker, J.M. 2003. *Victorian Soundscapes.* Oxford: Oxford University Press.
Pickering, D. 1972. Clicks, Whoops and Honks. *Archives of Disease in Childhood* 47:731–4.
Pinch, T. and K. Bijsterveld. 2004. Sound Studies: new technologies and music. *Social Studies of Science* 34(5):635–48.
Pinch, T. and K. Bijsterveld (eds). 2012a. *The Oxford Handbook of Sound Studies.* Oxford and New York: Oxford University Press.
Pinch, T. and K. Bijsterveld. 2012b. New Keys to the World of Sound. In *The Oxford Handbook of Sound Studies* (eds) T. Pinch and K. Bijsterveld, 3–35. Oxford and New York: Oxford University Press.
Pinch, T. and D. Reinecker. 2009. Technostalgia: how old gear lives on in new music. In *Sound Souvenirs: audio technologies, memory and cultural practices* (eds) K. Bijsterveld and J. van Dijck, 152–66. Amsterdam: Amsterdam University Press.
Pinch, T. and F. Trocco. 2002. *Analog Days: the invention and impact of the Moog synthesizer.* Cambridge, Massachusetts: Harvard University Press.
Pink, S. 2009. *Doing Sensory Ethnography.* London: Sage.
Porcello, T. 2004. Speaking of Sound: language and the professionalization of sound recording engineers. *Social Studies of Science* 34(5):733–58.
Porter, R. 1997. *The Greatest Benefit to Mankind: a medical history of humanity from antiquity to the present.* London: Fontana.
Reed, A. 2004. *Papua New Guinea's Last Place: experiences of constraint in a postcolonial prison.* Oxford and New York: Berghahn Books.
Reiser, S.J. 1978. *Medicine and the Reign of Technology.* Cambridge: Cambridge University Press.
Reiser, S.J. 1993. Technology and the Use of the Senses in Mid Twentieth-Century Medicine. In *Medicine and the Five Senses* (eds) W.F. Bynum and R. Porter, 262–73. Cambridge: Cambridge University Press.
Reiser, S.J. 1997. The Science of Diagnosis: diagnostic technology. In *The Companion Encyclopedia of the History of Medicine* (eds) W.F. Bynum and R. Porter, 826–51. New York: Routledge.
Revill, H. 2000. Music and the Politics of Sound: nationalism, citizenship and auditory space. *Environment and Planning* 18:597–613.

Rice, T. 2003. Soundselves: an acoustemology of sound and self in the Edinburgh Royal Infirmary. *Anthropology Today* 19(4):4–9.

Rice, T. 2005. Getting a Sense of Listening: a review of Michael Bull and Les Back (eds) *The Auditory Culture Reader. Critique of Anthropology* 25(2):199–206.

Rice, T. 2007. Listening as Touching and the Dangers of Intimacy. *Earshot: Journal of the UK and Ireland Soundscape Community* 5:15–21.

Rice, T. 2008a. Sound and the Boundless Body. In *Transplant* (ed.) V. Hume, 41–4. London: rb&hArts.

Rice, T. 2008b. The Doctor. *Erotic Review* 86:74–8.

Rice, T. 2008c. 'Beautiful Murmurs': stethoscopic listening and acoustic objectification. *Senses & Society* 3(3):293–306.

Rice, T. 2010. The hallmark of the doctor: the stethoscope and the making of medical identity. *Journal of Material Culture* 15(3):287–301.

Rice, T. 2012. Sounding Bodies: medical students and the acquisition of stethoscopic perspectives. In *The Oxford Handbook of Sound Studies* (eds) T. Pinch and K. Bijsterveld, 298–319. Oxford and New York: Oxford University Press.

Rice, T. 2013. Broadcasting the Body: the 'private' made 'public' in a hospital soundscapes. In *Music, Sound, and Space: transformations of public and private experience* (ed.) G. Born, 169–85. Cambridge: Cambridge University Press.

Richardson, R. 1987. *Death, Dissection and the Destitute.* London and New York: Routledge and Kegan Paul.

Rodaway, P. 1994. *Sensuous Geographies: body, sense, and place.* New York: Routledge.

Roseman, M. 1991. *Healing Sounds from the Malaysian Rainforest: Temiar music and medicine.* Berkeley, Los Angeles and London: University of California Press.

Rousseau, G.S. 2003. Introduction. In *Framing and Imagining Disease in Cultural History* (eds) G.S. Rousseau, M. Gill, D. Haycock and M. Herwig, 1–38. London: Palgrave Macmillan.

Roy, D.L. 2009. *The Pediatrician and Cardiac Auscultation.* Unpublished manuscript.

Sacks, O. 1989. *Seeing Voices: a journey into the world of the deaf.* Berkeley: University of California Press.

Salomon, B. 2001. On Being a Doctor: what the stethoscope said. *Annals of Internal Medicine* 135(1):56–7.

Samuels, D.W., L. Meintjes, A.M. Ochoa and T. Porcello. 2010. Soundscapes: toward a sounded anthropology. *Annual Review of Anthropology* 39:329–45.

Sartre, J.-P. [1943] 2002. *Being and Nothingness: an essay on phenomenological ontology* (trans. H.E. Barnes). London: Routledge.

Sawday, J. 1995. *The Body Emblazoned: dissection and the human body in renaissance culture.* London, Routledge.

Schaeffer, P. 1966. *Traité des Objets Musicaux.* Paris: Editions du Seuil.

Schafer, M.R. 1977. *The Tuning of the World.* New York: Knopf.

Schwartz, H. 2012. Inner Ear and Outer Sancta: earplugs and hospitals. In *The Sound Studies Handbook* (eds) T. Pinch and K. Bijsterveld, 273–97. Oxford and New York: Oxford University Press.

Segall, H.N. 1976. Autoauscultation in a Patient with Floppy Mitral Valve Syndrome. *American Heart Journal* 91(2):269–72.

Sennett, R. 1996. *Flesh and Stone: the body and the city in western civilisation.* New York and London: Norton.

Serematakis, N.C. 1994a. The Memory of the Senses, Part I: marks of the transitory. In *The Senses Still: perception and memory as material culture in modernity* (ed.) N.C. Serematakis, 1–18. Chicago and London: University of Chicago Press.

Serematakis, N.C. 1994b. Implications. In *The Senses Still: perception and memory as material culture in modernity* (ed.) N.C. Serematakis, 123–45. Chicago and London: University of Chicago Press.

Sharp, L.A. 2000. The Commodification of the Body and its Parts. *Annual Review of Anthropology* 29:287–328.

Shindler, D.M. 2004. Hand-held Ultrasound and the Stethoscope. *US Cardiology Online.* http://www.touchcardiology.com/articles/hand-held-ultrasound-and-stethoscope. Accessed 11/01/10.

Sinclair, S. 1997. *Making Doctors: an institutional apprenticeship.* Oxford and New York: Berg.

Smith, B.R. 1999. *The Acoustic World of Early Modern England.* Chicago: University of Chicago Press.

Smith, B.R. 2003. Tuning into London c.1600. In *The Auditory Culture Reader* (eds) M. Bull and L. Back, 127–36. Oxford: Berg.

Smith, B.R. 2004. Listening to the Wild Blue Yonder: the challenges of acoustic ecology. In *Hearing Cultures: essays on sound, listening and modernity* (ed.) V. Erlmann, 21–41. Oxford: Berg.

Smith, M.M. 2001. *Listening to Nineteenth-Century America.* Chapel Hill: University of North Carolina Press.

Smith, M.M. (ed.) 2004. *Hearing History: a reader.* Athens and London: University of Georgia Press.

Snow, C.P. 1964. *The Corridors of Power.* Kelly Bray: Stratus Books.

Soderquist, D.R. and J.W. Lindsey. 1972. Physiological Noise as a Masker of Low Frequencies: the cardiac cycle. *Journal of the Acoustic Society of America* 52:1216–20.

Sterne, J. 2003a. *The Audible Past: cultural origins of sound production.* Durham and London: Duke University Press.

Sterne, J. 2003b. Medicine's Acoustic Culture: mediate auscultation, the stethoscope, and the autopsy of the living. In *The Auditory Culture Reader* (eds) M. Bull and L. Back, 191–217. New York: Berg.

Stoller, P. 1989. *The Taste of Ethnographic Things: the senses in anthropology.* Philadelphia: University of Pennsylvania Press.

Stoller, P. 1997. *Sensuous Scholarship.* Philadelphia: University of Pennsylvania Press.

Sullivan, L. 1986. Sound and Senses: towards a hermeneutics of performance. *History of Religions* 26(1):1–33.

Supper, A. 2012. The Search for the 'Killer Application': drawing the boundaries around the sonification of scientific data. In *The Oxford Handbook of Sound Studies* (eds) T. Pinch and K. Bijsterveld, 249–70. Oxford and New York: Oxford University Press.

Taussig, M. 1992. *The Nervous System.* London and New York: Routledge.

Thompson, E. 2004. *The Soundscape of Modernity: architectural acoustics and the culture of listening in America, 1900–1933.* Cambridge, Massachusetts and London: MIT Press.

Tonndorf, J. 1972. Bone Conduction. In *Foundations of Modern Audition Theory* (ed.) J.V. Tobias, 206–235. New York: Academic Press.

Toop, D. 2010. *Sinister Resonance: the mediumship of the listener.* New York: Continuum.

Truax, B. (ed.) 1978. *The World Soundscape Project's Handbook for Acoustic Ecology.* Vancouver, British Columbia: ARC Publications.

Truax, B. 2001. *Acoustic Communication.* Westport, Connecticut and London: Ablex Publishing.

Turnbull, C. 1961. *The Forest People.* London: The Reprint Society.

Tyler, S. 1984. The Vision Quest in the West, or What the Mind's Eye Sees. *Journal of Anthropological Research* 40:23–40.

Valente, J.M., B. Bahan and H.-D. Bauman. 2011. Sensory Politics and the Implant Debates. In *Cochlear Implants: evolving perspectives* (eds) R. Paludneviciene and I.W. Leigh, 245–58. Washington: Gallaudet University Press.

Warren, R.M. 1982. *Auditory Perception: a new synthesis.* New York: Pergamon.

Watson, A. and D. Keating. 1999. Architecture and Sound: an acoustic analysis of megalithic monuments in prehistoric Britain. *Antiquity* 73:325–36.

Weiner, J. 1991. *The Empty Place: poetry, space and being among the Foi of Papua New Guinea.* Bloomington: Indiana University Press.

Wells, H.G. [1914] 1997. *The Country of the Blind and other Science Fiction Stories.* Mineola, New York: Dover Publications.

Welsby, P.D., G. Parry, and D. Smith. 2003. The Stethoscope: some preliminary investigations. *Postgraduate Medical Journal* 79:695–98.

Whitehouse, A. 2006. An Anthropologist Listens to Birds. http://www.st-andrews.ac.uk/soundanth/work/whitehouse/. Accessed 14/01/2012.

Wynne, J. 2007. Confidential Incident Report. *Static.* Issue 6. http://static.londonconsortium.com/issue06.

Yost, W.A. 1994. *Fundamentals of Hearing: an introduction.* San Diego: Academic Press.

Miscellaneous Websites

Heartbeat Babes. http://heartbeatbabes.com. Accessed 30/08/2011.

Filmography

Newell, M. 2007. *Love in the Time of Cholera.* 20th Century Fox.

INDEX

Ackerman, D. 96, 150, 177
acousmatic listening 42
acoustemology 53–71 *passim*
acoustic archaeology 11–12, 171
acoustic ecology 11, 93
acoustic illumination 70–1, 163, 179
acoustic objectification *see* objectification
acoustic perspective 3, 21, 30–1, 125, 141
agency 18, 40, 53, 74, 81, 88, 91, 119, 135, 154, 167–8, 183
amplification 19, 28, 50, 52, 65, 103, 105, 112–13, 115, 130, 139–40, 145, 150, 177, 180
anatomy 5, 55–6, 62–4, 66, 68, 78–80, 90, 134, 141, 151, 162, 165, 179
Anthony 31–4
apprenticeship 8, 10, 16, 68
audiovisual litany 117–19, 155, 169–70
auditory attention 1–2, 15, 19, 27, 42, 67, 80, 114, 173, 177, 181
auditory culture 94–5, 172–4
auditory focus 74, 103, 125
auditory knowledge 1, 4–5, 10–11, 16, 18, 48, 57, 70, 92–115 *passim*, 168
auditory space 12, 40–1, 43, 48–9, 51–3, 105, 137
Auenbrugger, L. 58–61, 64
aural body 177–81
auscultation *passim*; see also auto-auscultation, immediate auscultation, mediate auscultation
authority 4, 17, 19, 21–2, 32–4, 47, 65, 69, 82, 87, 95, 99, 153–4, 158–61, 163, 174–5, 183
auto-auscultation 19, 128, 137–52 *passim*, 180–1
autobiographical objects 88–9

Back, L. vii, 14, 32
background sounds 25, 37, 103, 107–8, 111
bells 12, 21–2, 33–4, 63, 109
Bentham, J. 22, 32
Berger, J. 5, 134, 165
Berendt, J. 119–20
Bijsterveld, K. vii, 71, 173, 181
biographical objects 88–9
body-as-self 131, 151
body techniques 96, 98, 114
Born, G. vii, 54
Bourdieu, P. 73, 78, 80, 95, 149, *see also* habitus, hexis
Bull, M. 12, 14, 32, 105
Brown, R. 177–80

captive audience 31, 38
cardiorotica *see* eroticism
Carpenter, E. 118, 177
'celebrity' patients 129–30
Chion, M. 98, 102
Chuengsatiansup, K. 9, 36–7
Classen, C. 9, 41, 57, 118
Clifford, J. 14–15
Corbin, A. 12, 21–2, 33–4, 52
Coltart, J. vii, 4–5, 16, 60–2, 75–7, 83, 87, 96, 98–100, 102–5, 107–9, 116, 123–5, 131–2, 140–2, 144, 148, 159, 163, 165–7, 178
contamination 44–5
conversation vii, 16, 30, 38, 45–8, 103, 129, 141, 165–7, 169, 175–6
Cusick, S. 39, 42, 53
cyborgs 52, 80

Dave 6, 102, 140–1
deafness *see* hearing impaired
Diane 6, 88
discipline 14, 22–4, 30, 32–3, 35, 57, 100
discursive space 17, 40, 45–8, 52, 180
display *see* stethoscope, display of
dispositions 73, 78–80, 90, 154, 182
dissection 55, 63, 68, 78–80, 90, 134, 141, 162
docile bodies 35, 182
doctor habitus *see* habitus
Downey, G. 105, 114
Duden, B. 139, 149, 163
Draper, J. 143, 149–50, 162
dys-appearance 139, 149–50, 181

ears 4, 14–16, 25–6, 45, 51, 53, 62, 68, 96, 100–2, 110, 120, 126, 143, 150, 177, 180, 187–8
echocardiograph/echocardiography 19, 49–53, 70, 86, 114, 137, 145, 148, 151, 153–70 *passim*, 180; *see also* ultrasound
Edinburgh Royal Infirmary 1, 4, 31, 34–6, 40, 42–3, 156, 175
electrocardiography/electrocardiograms/ECG 21–2, 25–7, 30, 35–6, 49–53, 70, 132, 137, 145, 148, 151, 161, 180
embodiment 6, 10, 13, 16–17, 37, 44, 73, 79, 91, 95, 138–9, 150, 181–2
ensounded(ness) 138, 179
Erlmann, V. 11, 14–15
eroticism 131–5, 138
ethnographic ear 14–17, 176
ethnographies of sound 11, 94

Feld, S. vii, 10, 15, 57, 65, 93–6, 108
Fleming, P. 57, 62, 68
Foi 10, 93–4
Foucault, M. 14, 17, 21–5, 32–3, 35, 55–6, 65, 70, 121–2, 126, 162–3, 182

Gallagher, M. 23–5, 28, 30
gaze 14, 23–4, 32, 39, 55–6, 70, 101–2, 117–18, 126, 131, 135, 141, 162–3
Gell, A. 10, 74, 81, 91, 93–6, 108, 118–19, 162
Gordon 41–2
Guy's Hospital 4–5, 68, 120–1

habitus 18, 73–4, 77–8, 80, 82, 88, 90, 92–3, 95, 114, 170, 182, *see also* dispositions
Haraway, D. J. 52, 80, 87
Harjit 6, 102, 140, 142
headspace 43, 53
hearing-impaired 11, 18, 95, 110–12, 154, 180
Heartbeat Babes 132–5
heart murmur *see* murmurs
Henriques, J. 138–9, 149, 177
hexis 94–5, 114, 139, 149–50
Hippocrates 57–8, 61, 188
Hooke, R. 58
Howes, D. 6–8, 10

immediate auscultation 57–8, 61–2, 131–2
Ingold, T. vii, 7–8, 137–8, 179
institutions, institutionalization 10–12, 20, 22–3, 30, 33–5, 37, 39–40, 44, 53–4, 73, 121, 173–4, 179–80, 183
intimacy 18, 40, 46, 53, 61, 66, 69, 87, 90, 117–18, 120, 125, 131–3, 165–6, 169, 178, 188
iStethoscope 105, 115, 173

Jackson, J. 120, 126, 128, 135
James 35–6
Jonse, Major General

Kaluli 10, 15, 57, 65–6, 93–6
Kirsch 72, 154, 169–70

Lachmund, J. 57, 66, 68–9
Laennec, R. 61–70, 72, 77, 109, 131, 162, 177
Latour, B. 68, 80–1, 158
Leder, D. 139, 150, 181
Lewis, G. 120, 126, 135
listening again 16, 116
listening-in-readiness 25, 27

Marks, G. 66, 82
Mary 6, 102, 141
Mauss, M. 94–5
mediate auscultation 17, 56, 62–4, 66, 131
medical anthropology 9–10
medical aurality 18, 57, 64
medical gaze 56, 70, 134, 162–3
medical habitus *see* habitus
medical school 5, 72–3, 78–80, 92, 141, 164, 167, 185

medical training 5, 72–4, 78–9, 90, 114, 121, 141, 160, 182
Mol, A. 50–1, 69, 151, 180
monitory listening 1, 17, 21–2, 24–9, 31, 70, 172, 181–2
murmurs 3, 29, 75, 97–9, 102–10 *passim*, 113, 116–17, 124–30 *passim*, 139–60 *passim*, 164–5, 167, 178, 185

Necker Hospital 62–3, 77
Nightingale, F. 28, 171
Nirit 110–15
nostalgia 165–6, 169–70
nurses 1, 4, 17, 21–39, 38, 45, 49, 51, 70, 76, 82–4, 86, 105, 121, 132, 172, 179–82

objectification 8–9, 14, 18–19, 46, 65, 116–36 *passim*, 152, 155, 166, 180
objectivity 46, 65, 69, 110, 116–18, 126–7, 152, 155, 158, 160–1, 163, 168–70, 176
olfaction 6, 9, 105, 119
onomatopoeia 93, 108–9
Osler, W. 146–7

panaudicism 22, 31, 33
panauralism 24, 26, 33
panopticism, Panopticon 14, 17, 21–6, 32–3, 35
patienthood 22, 35, 183
patient selves 17, 22, 35, 73
percussion 58, 60–1, 70
Porter, R. 59, 165
privacy 17, 26, 30, 38–9, 41–2, 44–5, 48, 52–3, 99, 130–1, 180
professionalization 12, 18, 57, 80

quiet 28–31, 34, 53, 100, 139, 141, 144, 149–50, 180

Reiser, S. 58, 62, 70, 160–1
Rhydd 110–11
Richardson, R. 55, 121–2
Rishi 6, 84–6, 88–9, 142–3, 159

St Thomas' Hospital vii, 1, 4–5, 18, 26, 28–9, 36, 40, 43, 46–9, 52, 72–3, 75, 82–3, 86, 89, 99, 105, 107, 109, 111, 115, 120–2, 128, 140, 144, 153, 159, 164, 168, 172, 175
Salomon, B. 88–9
Sartre, J.-P. 32–3
Sawalha, Nadia 76–7
Schaeffer, P. 42, 102
Schafer, M.R. 12, 135
Science and Technology Studies (STS) 13
Segall, H.N. 146–7
self-surveillance 29–30, 45, 53; *see also* surveillance
sensorial anthropology 6, 9
sensory politics 19–20, 153–5, 163, 169–70
Serematakis, N. C. 8–9
sexualization 117, 131–5, 184–8
Shindler, D. 105, 168

silence 29, 69, 145, 174
Sinclair, S. 60, 73–5, 78–80, 90, 92–3, 110, 142, 182
sleep 9, 25, 30, 37, 39, 43, 132–3, 143, 148, 188
sonic body 138–9, 177
sonic meaning 7, 20, 174
soundscape 11–12, 22, 25, 29, 31, 35–49 *passim*, 55, 65, 93–4, 137, 150, 172–3, 177, 179–80, 183
sound studies 11–14, 173
Sterne, J. 12–13, 62, 64–5, 68–9, 96, 111, 117–19, 155, 169–70
stethoscope *passim*; *see also* amplification
  as symbol 67, 73–4, 77, 82–3, 85, 90, 155, 166, 168–9, 183
  display of 71, 82–3, 90, 94, 168, 170
  death of 114, 154–5, 163–70, 183
  design of 66–7, 74, 84–5, 173
Stoller, P. 7–8, 10, 57, 118–19
succussion 57–8
Sue Ann 6, 75–7, 81
surveillance 17, 21–37 *passim*, 40, 45, 53, 140, 174, 181–2; *see also* panaudicism, panauralism

technoscepticism 166–8
Tom 6, 75–7, 80–1, 87–8, 102, 130, 140, 142
Truax, B. 25, 27
TV 32, 48, 75–7

ultrasound 13, 19, 49–50, 70, 86, 114, 149–50, 153–4, 157, 159, 161–4, 167, 173; *see also* echocardiography
Umeda 10, 93–4, 100, 162
unbounded body 48, 52, 180

visual evidence 8, 19, 161–2
visualism 14, 119

Wynne, J. vii, 38

X-ray 161, 167–8

Zafer 42–4
zones, zoning 8, 12, 17, 40, 45–8, 53, 111

www.ingramcontent.com/pod-product-compliance
Ingram Content Group UK Ltd.
Pitfield, Milton Keynes, MK11 3LW, UK
UKHW020816290926
15470UKWH00003B/1182

9 781907 774249